STOP BEING TOXIC

HOW TO QUIT NARCISSISTIC AND MANIPULATIVE BEHAVIORS, OVERCOME NEGATIVITY, AND BUILD HEALTHY RELATIONSHIPS

CHASE HILL

CONTENTS

A FREE GIFT TO OUR READERS

29 WAYS TO OVERCOME NEGATIVE THOUGHTS

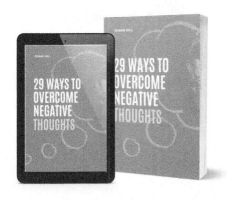

I'd like to give you a gift as a way of saying thanks for your purchase!

In 29 Ways to Overcome Negative Thoughts, you'll discover:

- 10 Strategies to Reduce Negativity in Your Life
- 7 Steps to Quickly Stop Negative Thoughts

- 12 Powerful Tips to Beat Negative Thinking

To receive your Free Ebook, visit the link:

free.chasehillbooks.com

Alternatively, you can scan the QR-code below:

If you have any difficulty downloading the ebook, contact me at **chase@chasehillbooks.com**, and I'll send you a copy as soon as possible.

INTRODUCTION

Have you ever wondered why others see your confidence, charm, and amazing skills as negative? Is it really that wrong to chase your dreams and strive for what you deserve? Do people actually confuse this with narcissism? Why is it acceptable for one person to have these personality traits while others are labeled for them?

The truth is, for many people, all of these qualities are excellent and highly beneficial, even greatly encouraged. So the question is, where is the line drawn?

A full-blown narcissist won't seek help, and they certainly wouldn't pick up a book like this for the simple fact that they can't see any problem with their personality or behavior. So the better question is, what does this say about you?

If we are completely honest with ourselves, we all either have a little toxicity in us or the potential of it. However, someone who is willing to self-reflect and work on their flaws may have narcissistic traits, but this is not the same as a narcissist who will manipulate anyone to get their way.

Before we delve into this topic in more detail, take a moment to give yourself some credit and appreciate that you have taken the first crucial step that many won't be able to do in their entire lives. You may not be perfect (who is?), but you aren't a bad person.

It's easier said than done, isn't it? All around you, relationships seem to be falling apart. Conflict is a daily occurrence, and it's impossible to decipher where all this hostility is coming from. Those closest to you may have tried to explain their point of view, but it feels like they are speaking in a foreign language and seeing things from a perspective far different from yours.

One of the hardest things for a person in your situation is to look in the mirror and see the reflection of a person that others don't see. In an argument, someone else may address one of your issues, but you may not see it in the same way. A textbook narcissist would dismiss these external opinions, but for you, it's confusing, even frustrating, and you are left wondering what you are missing.

What's even more infuriating is feeling like you're missing something that others seem to grasp easily. Since you're clearly intelligent, it's not just about their words, but their actions give a lot away. All of this leaves you feeling disconnected and isolated from others.

Thoughts start to spin out of control, and it doesn't matter how many times you replay an incident, you can't imagine how your words or actions could have played such a significant role. Anger starts to build up, and the cycle becomes a continuous loop.

The root cause of anger is often injustice, including the feeling of unfairness or wrongdoing. However, in your situation, the root cause of your anger stems from the frustration of not understanding, feeling pain, and being afraid. At this stage, it's hard to see this, but your toxic behaviors and narcissistic traits are deeply rooted in the fear of appearing weak, vulnerable, and not being good enough. As a result, you overcompensate as a defense mechanism to protect your self-esteem.

Even if you feel you have pushed your loved ones away, they will still be there to support you, but probably on one condition. You have to be accountable, own up to your flaws, and take those steps to make positive changes in your life.

Only you can commit to this, but there is a shining beacon of hope and help to keep you committed. *Stop Being Toxic* takes a fresh approach to removing those personalities holding you back. It's not about sugar-coating things or providing temporary quick fixes. It's about deep exploration that may even feel more painful at first, but the darkness starts to clear, and the changes will last a lifetime.

I have dedicated a significant part of my life as a coach and social interaction specialist to unraveling the complexities of the human mind and behavior. If there is one thing that stands out above the rest, it is that it's a journey of self-discovery, whether you are dealing with a toxic person or you are the toxic person. As you work through the process, you will embark on challenges as you uncover things about yourself that you would never have considered before. Each challenge you overcome will provide you with personal growth, meaningful relationships, and a more positive life.

Through my work, I have encountered some of the most incredibly toxic people. The combination of more than ten years of research and working with people who were determined to change their ways enabled me to come up with proven strategies that have opened pathways and opportunities. These strategies, which incorporate mental attitude, emotional resilience, and assertiveness, are going to be the foundations of your transformation.

With them, you won't just underpin the manifestations of your toxic behavior. You will also develop a greater sense of personal well-being as you learn to empathize, communicate, and master your emotions. Best of all, this journey doesn't end when you close this book. It's a transformation that will last a lifetime.

Before diving into these empowering strategies, let's begin our journey of self-reflection by discovering exactly what we are dealing with in terms of narcissism and toxic behavior.

CHAPTER ONE: MORE THAN JUST VANITY

> *I tell you, my dear, Narcissus was no egoist... he was merely another of us who, in our unshatterable isolation, recognized, on seeing his reflection, the one beautiful comrade, the only inseparable love...*

> *TRUMAN CAPOTE*

In Greek mythology, Narcissus was a hunter known for his attractiveness. He turned away the advances of all women, as the goddess of revenge, Nemesis, claimed it would be impossible for Narcissus to love anyone who fell in love with him.

One day, when leaning into a pool of water for a drink, Narcissus fell in love with his reflection. He was so drawn to his own beauty that he couldn't leave his reflection, and upon realizing that his love couldn't be reciprocated, his body melted away by the burning flames of passion inside.

Unfortunately, Greek mythology simplifies the complexities of narcissism today, and as Capote noted, it's not just about being a selfish person. The word narcissist is thrown around too liberally today, so before we get started, it's crucial to understand the difference between having narcissist traits and being a narcissist.

WHAT REALLY IS NARCISSISM?

When you hear the word narcissist, you picture a person who has an overly inflated ego and is self-centered. They need to be the focus of attention, especially in terms of recognition and praise. While this can provide a general description, there are different types of narcissism, and behaviors can vary between individuals.

Overt Narcissism

This is the most common view of narcissism. A person is incredibly outgoing to the point of being overbearing. They have a sense of entitlement and will exploit others to get what they want. They need praise, and this often makes them compete for admiration.

An overt narcissist is arrogant and tends to feel good about themselves. They often overestimate their abilities, intelligence, and emotional intelligence. This is especially true when it comes to how they avoid uncomfortable emotions and lack empathy.

Covert Narcissism

This type is also known as closet narcissism because the traits don't align with the usual perception of a narcissist.

These people seem to possess low self-esteem, lack self-confidence, and an introverted nature. They have a habit of playing the victim or being defensive, and criticism will be hard for them to accept because they will take it personally.

One study showed a link between covert narcissism and higher neuroticism, the tendency to experience uncomfortable and unpleasant emotions (Miller et al., 2017). This puts them at greater risk of anxiety and depression.

Antagonistic Narcissism

This is actually a subtype of the overt narcissist, where the person is more competitive and driven by rivalry.

They are still arrogant and will attempt to take advantage of others, but they are more prone to arguing and less likely to show forgiveness. Some antagonistic narcissists have a harder time trusting others.

Communal Narcissism

Communal narcissism is another subtype of overt narcissism and perhaps trickier to spot. Individuals with this trait have strong morals and intense reactions to anything they view as unfair.

They consider themselves to be empathetic and giving. While this doesn't seem like a bad thing, their own behaviors don't match the beliefs they feel so strongly about because they crave social power and a sense of importance.

Malignant Narcissism

As a severe form linked to overt narcissism, this type can cause serious problems in a person's life. They can have the same traits, such as the sense of grandiosity and need for praise, but it's often combined with vindictiveness and aggression. Some experience sadism (the enjoyment of others' pain) and paranoia. It's also possible for malignant narcissists to share traits with antisocial personality disorder. They can lack remorse, be reckless, and are more likely to have problems with money, the law, and substance abuse.

Even with a clearer understanding of narcissistic types, it's still not cut and dry. It's not a case of being an overt narcissist or a covert narcissist. A covert narcissist can have phases where overt narcissistic traits are more dominant and vice versa. At the same time, like most personality disorders, narcissistic traits lie on a spectrum, and it's not entirely negative!

For a long time, a lack of self-esteem, confidence, and self-love has been a huge problem for many. It's as if society went to the other extreme of narcissism, and it was seen as a bad thing to put our own needs above those of others. This is certainly true for parents who risk burnout in an attempt to balance work with their family responsibilities. Taking care of yourself is selfish when there is so much else to get done. We end up people-pleasing, unable to say no as we drown in responsibilities and ultimately feel like we aren't worthy of anything more. It's almost as if we fear standing up for ourselves and our needs in case we are wrongly labeled as narcissists.

The term "healthy narcissism" was coined by Paul Federn in the late 1920s and refers to a person's healthy self-love, which is necessary for creativity, empathy, confidence, and self-acceptance. Traits of healthy narcissism include:

- **Assertiveness:** The balance between passiveness and aggression in order to express needs and desires.

- **Self-love:** The ability to truly accept and love yourself while embracing strengths and areas for improvement.

- **Pride in abilities and achievements:** Recognizing that achievements require effort and hard work and appreciating the outcomes without boasting or trying to impress others.

- **Healthy boundaries:** Communicating boundaries shows self-respect and that you value your own time and resources.

- **Admiring others:** People have a healthy respect for others and their achievements without feeling threatened.

- **Goals:** Healthy narcissism includes having realistic goals and a solid plan to reach them. Self-awareness and confidence enable them to achieve their goals.

- **Compromise:** In a relationship, there is a balance of giving and receiving to ensure that both individuals' needs are fulfilled.

On the other end of the spectrum, narcissistic personality disorder (NPD) is a diagnosable mental health condition. Because people with NPD don't consider themselves to have a problem, it's difficult to know the prevalence, but different research has shown it to be as low as 0.5 percent of the general U.S. population (Ambardar, 2023) to up to 6 percent of the general population (Ronningstam, n.d.).

To be diagnosed with NPD, you need to meet five or more of the criteria outlined in the *DSM-5 (Diagnostic and Statistical Manual of Mental Disorders Fifth Edition)*. The criteria are:

- A grandiose sense of importance (exaggerates talants and achievements and expects to be recognized as superior even without achievements)

- Having fantasies of endless success, power, brilliance, beauty, or ideal love

- Requiring excessive admiration

- Having a sense of entitlement (refers to the belief that one deserves favorable treatment or that others should automatically comply with their expectations)

- Exploits others and takes advantage of others for their own gains

- Lacking empathy, unable to identify the needs and feelings of others

- Is often envious or thinks others are envious of them

- Shows arrogance, disdainful behaviors and attitudes

The major difference between having NPD and having narcissistic traits is that the traits a person suffering from NPD shows are consistent across all areas of their life. As mentioned before, at some point, we all have narcissistic moments. Who hasn't dreamed of the perfect partner or experienced a moment of road rage, expecting the other driver to back down? The above traits are fundamental to the personality of someone with NPD. What's more, these traits will have a significant negative impact on all areas of their lives, especially when it comes to relationships.

You are not a pathological narcissist! The main reason for this is that you have recognized your problems and need for change. Though these traits impact your life because they come and go, it doesn't feel like healthy relationships are impossible, and certain relationships may be more affected.

Because of the lack of self-awareness, it is impossible to self-diagnose NPD. Furthermore, NPD and narcissistic traits can overlap with symptoms of other mental health disorders such as bipolar disorder, PTSD, and antisocial personality disorder. If you are concerned about your traits and their impact on your life, please talk to a professional medical practitioner for support and guidance in managing symptoms.

From here on in, when we refer to narcissism, we will be discussing the traits rather than the diagnosable disorder.

ROOTS OF NARCISSISM

The exact cause of narcissism is unknown, and experts continue the nature versus nurture debate when trying to understand the development of such traits. In reality, narcissism is more likely a combination of genetics and biology (nature) and a person's environment and upbringing (nurture).

Let's clear one thing up: children aren't little narcissists despite any tendencies they may show. If you are a parent who is worried that your child's behavior is your fault, don't panic because it's never too late to make necessary changes. Children are naturally a little narcissistic as they learn about the world around them and their relationships. It is pretty common for a child to want to be the center of attention or seek more praise for their achievements. These normal behaviors in children are not signs that they will grow up to become narcissists.

That being said, childhood is an incredibly important stage for development, especially personality. It was once thought that narcissism was due to a lack of love and attention from parents, but it is now agreed that this isn't necessarily the case. Without placing all the blame on parents, let's begin with nurture.

While there are many parenting styles, there are three that can lead to a greater risk of narcissistic traits in adults. As originally thought, neglectful parenting may cause some children to develop narcissistic traits as a way to cope with parents being unresponsive to their needs. Their greater sense of self-importance may be a way of compensating for neglecting to validate thoughts and emotions. Abuse and maltreatment, whether emotional or physical, are high-risk factors.

An authoritarian parenting style may also encourage children to develop defense or coping mechanisms against feeling unloved or that they are never good enough. Strict rules and overcontrolling children push away the room for love, warmth, and open communication. The pressure parents put on children through high expectations may cause adults to chase endless dreams of success. It may also be possible that adults develop controlling behavior because it is what they were accustomed to during their upbringing.

On the other end of the scale, the indulgent parent may shower their child with love and praise, but often without justification. For example, if a 2-year-old puts their shoes on by themselves, they deserve a little celebration, a hug and kiss, and some words of encouragement. They don't deserve an expensive new toy.

If you are a parent who has had the fortune of watching *Bluey*, you may have seen the episode where one character tells his daughter that she is the most special girl in the world. Needless to say, the daughter breaks all the rules because she thinks she is special enough to get away with it. There is a difference between being special to you and being the most special. These inflated views can lead to children growing up assuming they are entitled.

The indulgent parent may also cave into rules that can manifest as weak boundaries. A child who has never learned how to establish boundaries isn't going to magically start as an adult. What's more, aside from not having their own boundaries, they will be more inclined to disrespect the boundaries of others.

Before giving your parents (or yourself if you are a parent) a hard time, remember that there is no one parenting style that has been concretely linked to narcissism, and it's not easy getting the right balance between love, boundaries, respect, motivation, and encouragement. Nevertheless, children mirror their parent's behavior, so if you feel like narcissistic traits run in your family, find peace in the fact that you can be the person to break that cycle.

Culture can also increase the risk of narcissism. There was a fascinating study on the differences between East and West Germany when the country was split after the Second World War. In West Germany, the culture was more individualistic compared with the collectivistic culture in East Germany. Results from an online survey showed that those in the former West Germany displayed higher levels of grandiose narcissism and lower self-esteem than those in the former East Germany. Yet, there was no difference in those who started school after the country reunited (Vater, 2018).

With regard to nature, certain narcissistic traits have been linked to genetics, specifically entitlement and grandiosity. NPD is one of the least studied personality disorders, so there is no certainty that these genetics are passed on to children.

Finally, in other cases, narcissistic traits may be due to a different brain structure. Brain scans carried out on people with NPD showed less gray matter in the brain (Jauk & Kanske, 2021). Gray matter density in the brain is associated with empathy. Other research has shown a link between NPD and increased levels of oxidative stress (Lee et al., 2020). Oxidative stress refers to the imbalance between free radicals and antioxidants in the body, and although this is biological, environmental factors can also lead to an increase in this imbalance.

Before you start to tell yourself that your narcissistic traits aren't your fault, which they may well not be, it's still important to hold yourself accountable for your actions today. To help with this, it's necessary to examine the extent to which these traits can impact your life.

THE RIPPLE EFFECT

A true narcissist can spend their entire life immune to the ripple effects of their behaviors. For two years, Emma and Oliver doted on each other, but Emma was heartbroken when she discovered Oliver was having an affair. He promised her it was over and proposed, assuring Emma that there was a future for the two of them. Each time after that, Oliver had the most perfect excuse that made Emma feel sorry for him. The ripple effect of Oliver's narcissism destroyed Emma's life, and it took years to regain any sense of self. However, Olivier continued as if nothing had happened, even questioning what he had done wrong when Emma finally left!

Oliver was a true narcissist. However, since you are not, the consequences of your actions will deeply affect most, if not all, areas of your life. Despite the image of grandiose and an exaggerated sense of self, at the core, you will probably feel shame, worthlessness, and possibly self-hatred. The drive for social status and to achieve goals may seem like the need for attention, but deep down, it's a way of avoiding fears, a lack of control, failure, and humiliation. After all, your narcissistic traits likely developed as a coping or defense mechanism. Regardless of overt or covert traits, your self-esteem is incredibly fragile.

In your relationships, you may find your angry outbursts are only exasperated, knowing that you are hurting your partner. Your empathy skills might not be as well developed as you like, but you can still see that they are in pain. But it's easier for you to ignore problems or avoid situations than to face your potential role in this. When conflicts arise, you may struggle to recognize facial expressions or emotions, which leads to feeling isolated in the relationship.

In the workplace, you may not notice how your need for praise and admiration leads to you taking credit for tasks and projects that others warranted credit for. It's hard for you to accept feedback, and it's possible you have gained a reputation for being arrogant, especially if you tend to overestimate your abilities. Again, the reality is that you don't genuinely feel like you are above criticism, but it's the fear of not feeling accepted that causes this.

Everybody's situation will be very different, but people with narcissistic traits can all relate to the sheer emotional turbulence they go through every day. Unfortunately, this is often something that others nearby don't understand. They may assume that as long as you are the center of attention, then you are okay.

The truth is that low self-esteem, the envy of others, and the lack of emotional regulation all contribute to an extreme sense of loneliness. Any attempt to explain how you are feeling comes out as an angry outburst rather than an expression of your sadness and anxiety.

Sadly, it's more than likely that your narcissistic behaviors don't just impact your life but also the lives of those around you. Please don't take this as a personal attack. As you read on, keep reminding yourself that you are here because you want to make a change. And part of this change is taking the time to consider the perspectives of others. Here are some ways narcissistic traits can cause ripple effects:

• Your partner may feel like you are using them in order to gain something, whether that's making others envious or having your needs met.

• It's likely that your partner feels that their boundaries are constantly being crossed.

• They might feel like they are always being lied to or

gaslighted, causing them to doubt their perception of reality.

- Your children might feel obliged to behave in a way that ensures your needs are catered to.

- They could feel as if their thoughts and feelings aren't valid or are being ignored.

- Colleagues are probably fed up with working in a toxic environment, walking on eggshells, and frustrated by your attitude.

- If you are in a position of authority, people may fear saying no to you, causing them to take on more than they can handle and impacting their health.

The ripple effect continues. The partner complains to their parents, and now the parents are worried. The child goes to school and picks on another child because they don't have the skills to process what is happening. The colleague goes home, and in the little time they have with their family, they are angry and frustrated.

In any type of relationship, both parties will find it hard to trust. From your point of view, trust is a challenge because opening yourself up can lead to disappointment. For other people, they just don't know what they are about to face at any given moment. I've seen friendships survive long distances and even couples without physical intimacy, but the hard truth is that no relationship can survive and flourish without trust. Vulnerability is the foundation of trust, and showing your weaknesses and true emotions can be simply terrifying!

Before your mind goes down the metaphorical and very dark rabbit hole, take a breath and remind yourself again that you are here for a change. While you will develop the ability to influence other people's emotions (without manipulating them), your first goal is to work on holding yourself accountable for your actions and emotions. Everything else will fall into place.

TIME TO SHIFT GEARS

How often have you heard that a leopard never changes its spots and that narcissists are incapable of change? Technically, this is not true because someone with narcissistic personality disorder doesn't see a reason to change. The next doubt to cross your mind is whether you are able to change, especially if you feel quite set in your ways.

It's easy to consider the brain the source of your problems, in particular, your negative view of the world, but in doing so, we overlook what a marvelous organ it really is. Did you know that during pregnancy, it was estimated that the average brain develops approximately 250,000 nerve cells per minute? (National Academies Press, 1992). It was once thought that the brain reached a certain age and stopped developing.

Today, we know that the human brain has around 86 billion nerve cells, or neurons (Caruso, 2023). These neurons receive information and communicate with other neurons by sending chemicals through a tiny gap called a synapse. It's estimated that a single neuron can have thousands of connections with other neurons, putting the total at over 100 trillion connections.

Imagine each of these connections as a muscle. The more it is used, the stronger the connection becomes. Neuro connections that aren't used or no longer needed eventually die, a process is known as synaptic pruning. This process of connections strengthening and weakening is called neuroplasticity, which means that anyone is capable of learning new things and changing.

Suppose you have a narcissistic trait of envy. Whenever you see someone with something you want, the neuro connections fire together, and your response is automatic. Replacing this thought with joy for the other person is hard at first because neurons need to make a new connection, but the more you practice this new strategy, the easier it becomes, especially as the "envy synapse" weakens.

I always find the science of neuroplasticity fascinating and reassuring. No matter what has happened in our past, there is a way to shift from the cloud of negativity to a life more positive.

Positivity isn't just about enjoying life with a smile on your face. A positive outlook leads to higher motivation and greater productivity. You become more resilient to tougher times and bounce back stronger. Stress and anxiety become easier to deal with and even less consuming as relationships become more fulfilling. Positivity is contagious, and your acts of kindness and gratitude have a knock-on effect on society!

To achieve this personal growth and increased life satisfaction, I have a straightforward yet highly effective REFLECT framework that guides you through seven steps to overcoming your narcissistic traits and leading a more positive, fulfilling life. We are going to:

- **R:** recognize toxic traits

- **E:** explore perspectives

- **F:** face your fears

- **L:** learn healthy patterns of interaction

- **E:** empathize with others

- **C:** cultivate positivity

- **T:** trust the process

Attempting to make this transformation on your own can leave you feeling more frustrated than before, especially without proven strategies. You are probably feeling that your narcissistic traits have already taken up too much of your life, so the last thing you want to do is waste time on anything that doesn't empower you.

This chapter has focused on narcissism, but there is more to toxic behavior than this. The next chapter will undoubtedly be challenging, but the first step is understanding what actually needs to change by discovering your toxic traits.

CHAPTER TWO: RED FLAG ALERT

> *Owning our story can be hard but not nearly as difficult as spending our lives running from it.*
>
> ## BRENÉ BROWN

In my experience, pain normally comes in one of two forms. There is the pain that blindsides you at the moment, like the sudden loss of a person, the end of a relationship, or losing a job.

The second type of pain follows us around, stemming from past experiences that we think we have dealt with but cause more damage than we realize.

Every painful moment caused by toxic traits adds to the pain that follows you around, and it makes running from the pain so much harder as if it's physically weighing you down.

Self-discovery and owning your story are indeed going to hurt, but it's a little like antiseptic cream—know that the pain is what will lead to healing.

As we embark on the first step of the REFLECT method, it's time to recognize toxic traits, some of which will be more obvious than others. But beyond this, we will also look at how to face these negative traits and even own them!

WHAT DOES TOXICITY LOOK LIKE?

Toxic traits are patterns of behavior that cause emotional harm, and the key word here is patterns. If someone makes a mistake, apologizes, and doesn't repeat it again, it's not the same as someone who continues to damage a relationship with the same behaviors. Narcissism is a form of toxic behavior, but not all toxic people have NPD.

However, like narcissism, toxic behavior often comes from a lack of self-awareness as well as insecurity, past trauma, or fears. Without self-awareness, people with toxic traits aren't aware of the pain they cause themselves or others.

Let's look at some of the most common toxic traits, and please bear in mind that they are not listed in any particular order.

Lying and Insincerity

Not telling the truth can be an outright lie or even the

omission of truth, and both can break the trust in a relationship.

Even if you begin with the truth, you may find yourself deviating from it. You may also feel compelled to tell lies to cover up previous lies.

Words can be insincere, but an insincere person is someone who isn't authentic. Examples include self-censoring during a conversation or craving attention over genuine connections. The roots of insincerity are often a fear of being vulnerable.

Example: Your partner asks about who you went out with, and you purposely leave out someone you have a history with.

People Pleasing

People pleasing is a toxic trait that causes harm to yourself more than others. This habit involves saying yes to doing things you really don't want to do and apologizing excessively even when you did nothing wrong.

It's also likely that you don't speak out or stand up for your beliefs and values for fear of repercussions. People pleasing also means that self-care is often neglected.

Example: You need a quiet weekend at home but your parents invite you for dinner. When you try to say no, your mom tells you that your siblings have all agreed.

Perfectionism

Toxic perfectionism can cause yourself and others pain because of unrealistic expectations and high standards. The need to be perfect can cause constant dissatisfaction and impossible levels of pressure. There is an intense fear of failure that comes with perfectionism.

Example: You spend 30 minutes obsessing over a 3-sentence email, writing and rewriting it, fearing that there might be a mistake or that the message will be misinterpreted.

Flexibility and Inflexibility

A person or a company with too much flexibility will struggle to stick to rules and structure, and there will be minimal clarity in their lives.

On the other end of the scale, inflexibility can come across as extreme rigidity with no give or take. Even when evidence to the contrary is presented, an inflexible person will still stand their ground.

Example: A flexible parent would let their teenage child stay out partying all night. An inflexible parent won't let their teenage child out without them.

Judging Others

Judging others is closely linked to another toxic behavior: comparison. You might find yourself comparing your actions, behaviors, achievements, and even things like morals and beliefs to those of others and judging the people who don't match your comparisons.

Essentially, this is a reflection of how you feel about yourself, and you might criticize the actions of others to validate your own decisions.

Example: You observe another parent and wonder why on earth they would let their child eat candy so close to dinner.

Competition

Similar to judging, unhealthy levels of competition only lead to comparing your life with others. While a small amount of competition can increase motivation, the need to win all the time takes the fun out of activities and creates tension with others. Competitiveness can be made worse by perfectionism.

Example: When you are playing games with your children, you never let them win, even when you see how discouraged they are.

Negative Self-Talk

There is a fine line between recognizing your flaws and falling into the trap of rumination. Because it's human nature to look on the negative side, it's easy to take a flaw and catastrophize it, making it worse than it could actually be.

The loop of negative self-talk can impact your sleep and mood, increasing anxiety. In turn, this can put added strain on relationships. With neuroplasticity in mind, replaying negative thoughts strengthens the connections to the point where your brain may actually begin to believe these untrue thoughts.

Example: Your friend is trying to give you some feedback, and they tell you one good thing and one thing to work on. You completely ignore the good feedback and replay the negative feedback in your mind until you convince yourself your friend must hate you.

Pessimism

Seeing the glass half empty can have a paralyzing effect for all involved. For you, it brings your morale down, possibly causing a defeatist attitude, such as telling yourself, "Why bother trying if it'll only end in failure and giving up sooner?"

A pessimistic outlook quickly rubs off on others, bringing them down too. Those looking to maintain their positive attitude may start to avoid you.

Example: You walk into an interview thinking you are going to mess up and not get the job despite your qualifications and experience.

Attention-Seeking

Excessive attention-seeking can involve catastrophizing events, making self-deprecating comments, or oversharing on social media just to get likes. People seeking attention may resort to making others feel uncomfortable, embarrassed, or irritated in order to get their attention.

Example: You post political memes on Facebook, knowing it will annoy your mother-in-law enough to get a response.

Manipulation

Manipulation is a form of influence in order to gain control, power, or personal benefit. Some manipulation is more obvious, such as lying, placing the blame, judging, or ridiculing others.

It can also be far more subtle, like knowing someone's weaknesses and taking advantage of them or encouraging people to give up meaningful relationships so that they depend more on you.

Example: You ask a team member to stay late to complete a task and explain it has to be them because nobody else would be able to do the job as well as they can.

Gaslighting

This is a form of emotional manipulation where you say things to confuse people and question their reality, even sanity. It often starts with smaller incidents but can often lead to the other person suffering from emotional abuse and isolation.

Comments that are a sign of gaslighting include "You're imagining things," "You're too sensitive," "You're overreacting," and "You're crazy."

Example: Your partner mentions how you were slightly rude to their sister, and you reply, "It's all in your head."

Playing the Victim

Someone who has a habit of playing the victim will always blame someone else for their problems and are unable to get themselves out of difficult situations. They tend to expect others to come to their rescue instead of trying to solve the issue on their own. This behavior is often accompanied by a lot of negativity and manipulation.

Example: You cheat on your partner but blame them because they were never around.

Guilt-Tripping

This is a form of manipulation where emotions are used as a way to control others, and guilt is an incredibly powerful emotion. People often feel guilty about their choices or actions, which can lead them to believe they are being selfish.

Example: Any phrase that involves "If you loved me, you would…" is a form of guilt-tripping another person to change.

The Dramatics

Drama is used as a way of seeking attention or gaining control. There are several ways a person can revel in the dramatics, but it's commonly through exaggerated stories, lies, rumors, or gossip. In some cases, the dramatist will start arguments. For others, the constant drama is draining.

Example: Your boss tells you something in confidence that is necessary for your role as a leader, but you can't resist telling others to show off your status of having "insider knowledge."

Holding on to the Past

Our pasts are good for wonderful memories and learning experiences. Hanging on to painful experiences and unresolved issues only causes you suffering and, by extension, those around you. Holding onto grudges is a sign of chronic unforgiveness!

Example: Your brother scratched your car ten years ago, and since then, you have never let him drive one of your cars.

Conversation Hogger

While this can also be about not giving others the chance to talk, it's more about ensuring the conversation is always about you. If someone starts telling you about a problem they have, you redirect the conversation back to your own issues. It's rare for you to ask other people questions during a conversation.

Example: Your partner starts telling you about their day, and you interrupt with things like "That's nothing compared to my day..." or "Wait until you hear about what happened to me..."

Clinging

Clinginess is subjective, so what one person feels is clingy could be different from the next. It refers to a constant need for reassurance or support, which is often observed in relationships. Even if your partner shows plenty of love and support, you may still feel insecure and fear being abandoned.

Example: You call your partner multiple times in a day and send numerous messages. When they don't reply, you start overthinking, convinced they are doing something wrong.

Control Freak

Being a control freak means having an obsessive need to be in charge of everything and everyone. You try to micromanage other people and their lives, which can be very suffocating for those around you. Control freaks will even try to manage situations that are out of their control or can't be changed.

Example: You insist on everything being done a certain way in the office, and when people don't follow your plan, you get moody, agitated, and snap at your coworkers.

Apathy

Someone suffering from apathy has a persistent absence of emotions and a sense of detachment from the world. Nothing seems to matter to you, whether that's spending time with people or your favorite pastimes. There is little enthusiasm for making plans or setting goals.

Example: You work in a job that requires empathizing with others, but you have recently noticed that you are feeling lethargic, which prevents you from connecting with others. Your supervisor warns you that if you can't find a way to regain your empathy, you will need to look for another job. But you don't even care about this warning.

Greed

Selfishness is a common trait of narcissists; however, greed is about wanting more than you need at the cost of others. Even when you gain more than you need, you won't feel satisfied. Greed can also be displayed through stinginess, such as refusing to share time or possessions.

Example: Despite being financially comfortable, you raise the rent of your tenant's rate without considering how this might affect them.

Love Bombing

In the early days of a relationship, love bombing is an excessive amount of affection and attention in order to manipulate a person into a relationship.

It's a form of emotional abuse that is difficult to recognize because the other person is receiving a boost of self-esteem and may not see the warning signs. Love bombing can involve the overuse of flattery, showering your new partner with unwanted and unnecessary gifts, and over-communicating feelings.

Example: You have been seeing someone for a couple of months, and they are your soulmate and the love of your life. You give them a key to your place and insist they move in because you couldn't possibly live another day without them.

Perspectives have to be taken into consideration here, which is a challenge if you don't feel like you can rely on your empathy skills.

In the instance of love bombing, one person might be more than comfortable with adorable messages every hour, but the next person could find this suffocating. At the same time, a random gift to show appreciation shouldn't be feared as a sign of love bombing.

This brings us back to the spectrum of traits. Everyone has moments of toxicity, whether that's a moment of greed when you really don't want to share your favorite dessert with your children or when you wake up one morning and everything looks sad and dreary.

It's when these traits become continuous and impact your daily life (like the traits of narcissism) that you need to take the necessary steps.

FACING THE TRUTH ABOUT YOURSELF

There is no point in feeling bad about yourself or getting frustrated. Having toxic traits doesn't make you an inherently bad person. Like many others, your behaviors are unintentional, and you might not even be aware of them. Everyone has negative traits, even the most successful people in the world. What makes all the difference is knowing exactly what the problem is before attempting to fix it. If any of the narcissistic or toxic traits sound familiar to you, it's now time to take responsibility for those actions.

Owning up to things is so much more complicated than it seems. It's like a trip down memory lane, waiting for someone to tell us off or punish us for our actions. Again, it's not about blaming the parents, but if you grew up in an atmosphere where apologies were forced, and mistakes were punished, it's normal not to appreciate the benefits of taking responsibility. As adults, taking responsibility for our actions also means acknowledging our flaws as human beings!

Taking responsibility isn't the same as blaming or looking for a scapegoat. It's about being responsible for your part in a situation or experience and, therefore, some responsibility for the outcome.

If you have ever been on a date and the person spends the entire time complaining about their ex, there are several red flags. First, they are stuck in the past and are portraying their ex as crazy without taking responsibility for their role. People don't act out for no reason. Your date may have had other toxic traits that caused their ex's behavior and, ultimately, the demise of the relationship.

Responsibility is crucial in relationships. If someone comes across as if they never make a mistake, it's impossible to relate to them and build bonds. If you can own up to your part in something, it enables others to see a little bit of themselves in you (the flawless human). On the contrary, by denying all responsibility, you can expect to create a barrier between other people as you seem less trustworthy. You will gain more respect by owning up to mistakes and moving on from them rather than hiding from them.

At the same time, these mistakes are ideal learning opportunities. Imagine not paying attention to your child's problem and having them come home from school the next day with even greater stress and trouble. It's an invaluable lesson that we can't ignore our responsibilities if we don't want our loved ones to suffer. It's part of your personal growth that will prevent smaller problems from escalating into bigger ones.

Finally, taking responsibility actually improves your decision-making skills. When we don't take responsibility, we can end up making self-justifications or excuses for our actions.

The harsh reality is that these self-justifications are distortions of the truth, and one can lead to another, firing off a domino effect. The information used to make decisions is now warped. To make the best choices in life, you need to ensure your information is accurate and without prejudices.

Some of the decisions you make will have a direct impact on those around you. Though making tough decisions can be challenging, it's unfair for others to delay or make choices based on inaccurate information.

Being responsible means you have the strength to make the best decisions, follow through with them, and admit if things don't go as planned so that adjustments can be made.

The only way you are going to fail in life is by not taking responsibility and action after making a mistake. It's scary but also quite liberating.

Here are some examples of how people can take responsibility.

● Accept that you are the driver of your life, not a passenger.

● You recognize your part in different situations, the good and the bad.

● You don't make excuses when things go wrong.

● You don't blame others for your part in things that have gone wrong.

● If you hurt someone with your words, you can genuinely apologize and take steps to improve your communication.

• You don't delegate your responsibilities to others.

• When things don't go well in your personal and professional life, you look for solutions rather than burying your head in the sand.

Knowing why you should take responsibility for your negative traits isn't quite the same as recognizing and fully owning them.

Let's take that one step at a time!

Step #1: Identify Your Negative Traits

Here is where self-reflection begins to kick in, and there is no rush to achieve this all at once. You may want to take a few days to make sure you have taken the necessary time to fully consider all of your negative traits. This can be done by journaling your thoughts, feelings, and actions.

The best way to get to the roots of your negative traits is to use the Why Technique and keep asking yourself why until you have a lightbulb moment that reveals a negative trait. For example:

My colleague doesn't want to work with me.

Why?

Last month there was a bit of a disagreement during a project.

Why?

They disagreed with my idea.

Why?

My idea may have been one-sided.

From here, I can see that one of my negative traits would be to assume I know better and not respect the input of team members.

Another way to discover more about your negative traits is to look at your triggers and what makes you react in ways you don't like. If you tend to lose your temper or go into a mood, consider who you were with and what you were doing before the change.

You may also want to journal this so you can keep track of patterns. Pay close attention to the things that irritate you in others because they are often a reflection of what we don't like about ourselves.It's always beneficial to get different perspectives on your negative traits by asking those you trust for feedback. Tell them you are looking for genuine personal growth, so you need them to be honest about any behavior you could change.

Step #2: Step Outside Your Traits

Once you have a list of traits, it's time to take a closer look at each one. Be blunt, and don't hold back as you write (or at least consider) a complete version of that trait. Imagine yourself as a bystander. What does your negative trait look like to them?

Step #3: Consider Those Around You

Next, take each of your negative traits and consider how they affect the people around you. Follow this up with how you feel, knowing that your behaviors are causing these secondary effects.

If you start to feel overwhelmed, take a break, but don't give up. Knowing how your behavior affects others and your own life will provide you with greater motivation to change.

Step #4: Monitor Your Traits

Real change takes knowledge and time, so don't try to rush the process and change everything all at once. At this stage, it's important to note every time negative traits arise and the reasons behind them. Keep as much detail as you can to increase your awareness. This can include times of the day, locations, and even how exercise and diet may impact your mood and behavior.

But what if you have done all this and still struggle to identify your negative traits? In that case, you may be troubled by blind spots!

SEEING THE UNSEEN

Blind spots refer to areas of your character that you are not aware of or don't know about yourself. As much as we like to think we know who we are, there are certain unknowns that are only visible to others, and you might have reached a point where others aren't completely comfortable being honest with you.

There are four types of blind spots, all related to assumptions or misjudgments:

1. Knowledge blindness: We think our cognitive abilities are higher than what they really are.

2. Beliefs bias: Also known as confirmation bias, this means we only believe information that supports our beliefs.

3. Emotional blindness: Our emotions cloud our view of reality and judgments.

4. Thoughts blindness: Like emotions, if you only look at things from your thoughts, your judgment will be clouded. What we think of ourselves isn't necessarily true.

Blind spots are going to vary from person to person. They will be greatly influenced by an individual's emotions as well as the person's character and the situation. Nevertheless, there are some common blind spots that people with toxic and narcissistic traits may suffer from:

• A lack of empathy

• Difficulty with feedback

• Overestimating one's abilities

• The expectation of special (unwarranted) treatment

• Intentional or unintentional manipulation

• Blaming relationship problems on others

The previously mentioned steps to identifying negative traits will increase self-awareness, and this, with time, will help uncover blind spots. This can happen faster when you take advantage of the Johari window.

The Johari Window, created by psychologists Joseph Luft and Harry Ingham, is a tool for understanding gaps in your reality and assumptions. The model is divided into four areas: the arena, the mask, the blind spots, and the unknown.

The Johari Window

	Known to Self	Unknown to Self
Known to Others	**Arena** (what you and other people know)	**Blind Spots** (what you can't see about yourself but others know)
Unknown to Others	**Mask/Facade** (what you share or hide about yourself)	**Unknown** (what you don't know about yourself and neither do others)

The goal of the Johari window is to expand the arena because this is the area that builds clarity and trust. And, as the arena area grows, the blind spots and the aspects you hide behind a mask are reduced.

The simplest way to do this is to start sharing more with others. This doesn't have to be all of your deepest, darkest secrets, but even gradually letting people in will make it more comfortable for both of you when it comes to asking for feedback, which, in turn, will reduce the blind spots. When these two things start to happen, what neither you nor others know about you becomes more clear!

Alternatively, you can record yourself to get to know yourself better. At first, you may find yourself more "on guard" as you are recording, but even then, this will still give you insights into your microexpressions, those you can't control, and how you react in different situations. The more information you can gather, the more objective you will become!

You can do a simple activity to expand the arena area of your Johari window. Begin by writing down five words that describe you. Now, ask nine other people to do the same, ensuring that three are friends, three are family members, and three are coworkers or from a different social setting to the first six. Let them know that the idea of the activity is to discover more about yourself, not to inflate your ego!

Once you have everybody's words back, start comparing the similarities and differences. What things do you like about yourself, and what words come under areas for improvement? It will be interesting to see if there are certain traits that are more apparent with different people, indicating how your behavior changes in different situations.

Don't forget to thank people for their efforts in helping you. It's not easy providing constructive criticism, especially not to someone who has been less than willing to accept it in the past!

As we move on to the next chapter, it's time to take the first step toward better empathy as we discover the wonderful advantages of seeing your own world through different lenses and perspectives.

CHAPTER THREE: LIFE IN HD

> *If you change the way you look at things, the things you look at change.*

DR. WAYNE DYER

How individuals view things can be quite fascinating! There are plenty of images on social media that explain just how different our perspectives can be. The image of the rabbit and the duck is a classic example, with some people seeing a duck first and others seeing the rabbit.

There are some images where, no matter how hard you look, you cannot seem to see the same image as another person. In this chapter, we will remove the rose-tinted glasses as we cover the E in the REFLECT framework and explore perspectives.

PERCEPTION VS. PERSPECTIVE

Your perception is the physical sensations you interpret as a result of observation. Your perspective is the mental view of your perceptions. Both contribute to the way you view the world and, essentially, your reality. Each person's perspective will differ due to many influencing factors involved. Understanding these factors is often enough to appreciate a newfound respect for other people's perspectives.

One of the biggest influences on our perspective is our past experiences. Imagine if two people went to a party, and one found it super boring while the other had a great time. The first person is likely to dread the next party, while the second would be more inclined to look forward to it.

Rather than reading through the following list, take a moment to think about each influencing factor and how your perception could be shaped:

- **Education:** The way individuals interpret and organize information varies based on their country and cultural background.

- **Expectations:** Your subconscious tells you what to look for. The brain has a habit of creating patterns of expectations that are hard to shut off.

- **Circumstances:** Circumstances provoke different expectations. Think about how you perceive an alleyway at night versus during the day.

- **Senses:** People's senses react definitely to stimuli. A blind person may hear things that the next person doesn't, just as someone who has a highly sensitive sense of smell will interpret information differently.

- **Age:** As we grow older, certain things become more or less important. As teens, your perspective on retirement will differ greatly from what it is as an adult.

- **Mood:** A tiny annoyance can either be seen as a huge issue or a walk in the park, depending on your mood.

- **Emotions:** Perceived negative or perceived positive emotions can influence how stimuli are interpreted.

- **Motivation:** We are more likely to notice things that interest us.

- **Personal beliefs and values:** How you view issues like equality, racism, politics, and religion can cause you to see things differently

- **Media:** The cultivation theory proposes that media can alter attitude and behavior of people.

Take the following image as an example of how easily perception can be influenced.

The Bruner and Minturn study consisted of two groups of students. One group was shown a series of numbers, and the other, a series of letters.

Afterward, both groups were shown an ambiguous figure.

B

The group that was shown the series of numbers viewed the figure as the number 13, whereas the group that was shown the series of letters saw the letter B. This may seem insignificant, but imagine how many images we are exposed to on a daily basis and how easy it is for others to shape our perspective.

It's our responsibility to broaden our own perspectives and ensure that we have all the necessary information not to allow others to negatively sway our perspectives.

THE POWER OF PERSPECTIVE

According to an Indian folk tale, there were once six old blind men living in a village. They spent ages debating what an elephant was like based on stories they had heard from others. Their opinions ranged from the magical to the terrifying, with one man claiming elephants didn't exist. Tired of arguing, they went to visit a palace one day where an elephant stood on the grounds.

Each blind man touched a part of the elephant and came up with further opinions. The elephant was like a wall, a snake, a spear, a cow, a carpet, and a rope. After more arguing, the palace owner interrupted and asked how each man was so certain they were right. Each man had only touched one part of the puzzle, and it wasn't until they put those pieces together that the truth about the elephant would be understood.

It's hard to imagine how many conflicts arise simply because one person is unable to see a different perspective. It can start with something so innocent, like the ambiguous figure and whether it's a B or a 13. But then the argument gets sidetracked, and other situations and emotions get dragged into the discussion. Before you know it, you have forgotten about the figure and are debating why you have to spend the holidays with your in-laws again.

Perspective is fundamental for learning, creativity, and problem-solving. Imagine having a problem and only having your knowledge and past experiences to solve it. As soon as you speak to one other person to gain their perspective, you have doubled your chances of finding a better solution.

It's important to consider whose perspectives you are also taking in. If you ask five white middle-aged businessmen for their perspectives, their viewpoints are likely to be relatively similar. Once you expand your scope and ask people from different age groups, cultures, and backgrounds, the perspectives become far more open and less biased.

Because your perspective determines your thoughts, which are directly related to your actions, having a diverse range of perspectives can help your communication and interactions immensely. Taking in such a range of information enables you to challenge your own and other's preconceived opinions, making biases more apparent. This openness leads to increased inclusion and equal access to opportunities, which improves society as a whole.

Perspectives give us firsthand experiences of the lives of others and their struggles. Speaking of senses and stimuli, people with neurodevelopmental disorders, such as autism or attention deficit hyperactivity disorder (ADHD), often have trouble with sensory processing. You may have heard about how some people find lights to be too bright or sounds to be too loud, but it's only when you actually listen to the perspective of these people that you can truly understand what their lives must be like. This is when empathy truly starts to develop.

A word of warning, though! In a world that desperately needs diversity, different perspectives, and empathy, technology is not always helpful when it comes to personal growth. If you have read any of my other books, you will know that I am not against technology. However, I am cautious of the potential downfalls, especially in our ability to communicate.

Aside from the media having the power to shape our perspectives, the more and more common use of personalized content can also limit our exposure to different perspectives. Whether it's streaming platforms or social media, algorithms suggest content to see based on our preferences, and unfortunately, this can often exclude anything that could cause discomfort. It's these uncomfortable things outside of our comfort zones that spark curiosity, learning, and acceptance.

The 'Recommended for You' feature is convenient, but every now and again, make an effort to scroll past these recommendations and explore new content to broaden your horizons.

A DIFFERENT VIEW

Expanding your perspectives is an excellent start. The more open-minded you are, the easier it will be for you to appreciate the perspectives of others, a process known as perspective taking or theory of the mind as we attempt to understand the mental states of others. This requires the activation of many areas of the brain as you set aside your own mindset and shift into the state of mind of someone else.

This isn't the same as mind reading or having a psychic connection. But as we have seen how perspective is unique, it does take a certain amount of cognitive capacity and emotional intelligence to intentionally distance your own perspective from that of others. To understand the perspective of others, you need to be able to consider their thoughts, feelings, and motives without judgment. This is an active process, unlike your own perspective, which is something automatic.

Perspective taking is highly beneficial because as you consider someone else's perspective, you start to see more of yourself in them. Imagine a coworker who had recently lost a parent. From an outside perspective, it is clear that this is a painful experience. But when you stop to reflect on what it feels like to go back home to a place where your loved one is no longer there, and you remember how it felt when you lost someone, there is a deeper connection that wouldn't have been established without perspective taking.

Nevertheless, there are a few barriers to perspective taking. Since your perspective is deeply ingrained and occurs naturally, you have to activate the ability to consider someone else's perspective. This has to be a deliberate action that takes time. Considering another person's perspective is more difficult and takes longer compared to considering your own point of view. You won't always have the complete information to understand another person's perspective, and our assumptions and inferences aren't entirely accurate.

During a conversation, there may already be a lot going on if you are working on active listening. If you can't take a moment to think about how a person is feeling or what they are thinking during an interaction, make a commitment to do so later on. You could even reach out to them through a phone call or message once you have thought about their point of view.

If you feel like you are missing a part of the picture or you need clarification, ask the person questions rather than assuming.

Let's finish up with some tips and exercises to improve perspective taking:

1. The Movie

Besides a movie, this exercise can be done with a book or a series. Choose one character, preferably someone you can relate to, as this will be easier to start with than someone whose perspective may differ greatly from yours. Also, fictional characters are easier to understand because you aren't as emotionally attached to them as you are to people in your life.

During the movie/show/book, pause a quarter of the way through and again halfway and three-quarters of a way through. Ask yourself what your character is thinking about at that point and why. Think about why they are behaving in a certain way and what emotions they could be experiencing.

When you have finished, ask yourself how well you understood the character and their actions. Could you see the events in a similar way to the character? Were you accurate in your emotional understanding?

2. Your Imagination

Take a photo or an image with at least two or three people. Don't make it an image where you know the people or a photo of a past experience; it has to be an unknown snapshot. Spend a few minutes writing down a story about what is happening in the image, including the lead-up and the outcome. Naturally, this is your perspective.

Next, spend a few minutes rewriting the story, but this time, from the perspective of one of the people in the image. Don't forget to consider what they might be thinking and feeling at that particular moment. Repeat the same process for other people in the image.

Once you have finished, take a few final minutes to think about whether you were able to differentiate between the perspectives. Because perspectives are so unique for each person, the narratives for each story need to be different.

3. Using Your Past Experiences

Think about a recent conflict you had. You can also write about it if this helps your brain process information better. Begin with one sentence summarizing the argument. Now, put yourself in the other person's shoes. How did the conflict play out in their mind? Write about what they were thinking and feeling, as well as how they perceived your words and actions during the conflict. Finish the activity by thinking about what you could have done differently but from the perspective of the other person. Don't worry if this one is a little more challenging and may require more patience with yourself and practice.

4. Role Reversal

For this, you will need a willing partner to switch roles with. Role reversal is a great exercise for creating empathy and understanding by stepping into someone else's shoes and experiencing things from their point of view firsthand.

Take, for example, a toxic couple where one partner comes home from work every night and spends a couple of hours on their hobby while the other partner is at home taking care of the children, helping with their homework, preparing dinner, and other chores. Role reversal would have the toxic partner stay at home while the other person would go out to enjoy themself. The toxic partner would have to take on the same chores as the other partner and appreciate the stress and hard work that they go through each night.

There is no end to the possibilities of role reversal. Doctors can be treated as patients, teachers become students, parents become the child, and so on. However, it's important that both people involved set guidelines and goals before initiating role reversal. It should be treated as a learning opportunity rather than a chance to throw blame and guilt at each other, so schedule time afterward for feedback and reflection.

5. Pre-Interaction Perspective Taking

Imagine you are about to meet someone for a coffee or step into a meeting. Before you open the door, take a brief moment to think about how the other person might be feeling at the same moment.

Reflect on their values, beliefs, and motives and how they can impact everything that is about to occur during your interaction. Be sure to practice this exercise with various relationships, such as colleagues and family members, and in different settings, even with the same person, but in other settings. Just like yours, their perspective will change depending on their environment.

Seeing things from another person's point of view is not easy, especially when there is a lot of history and painful emotions involved. It also requires putting one's ego aside. No matter how right you think you might be, it doesn't mean that other people aren't entitled to their own perspective. When you are able to see insights into this, your ego may even be a little bruised. That being said, the improvements in relationships will far outweigh the damage to your ego!

Seeing things as others may give you a glimmer of what they might be feeling because of your toxic traits, but it won't necessarily stop these behaviors. In the next chapter, we will embark on confronting and overcoming the fuel of your toxic behavior!

CHAPTER FOUR: FACE THE MUSIC

 Fear is not your enemy. It is a compass pointing you to the areas where you need to grow.

STEVE PAVLINA

Take a moment to consider what the most powerful emotion is.

If you scroll through forums, answers vary from lust to hope, but one that creeps up more frequently than others is fear.

Movie makers have profited from it, marketers have used it to influence buyers, and parents have manipulated children with it!

But is fear something that should be dreaded, or have we got our perspectives wrong?

WHAT IS FEAR EXACTLY?

I have always felt that understanding more about how emotions are formed is an essential step toward overcoming personal struggles, especially when it comes to fear. It is interesting to note that some of the same chemicals that lead to happiness and excitement are also used in the fight-or-flight response when we are exposed to a threat or fear. So, what makes fear such a powerful emotion?

Our senses pick up stimuli in the environment and send messages to the amygdala, a part of the limbic system, which is responsible for processing emotional stimuli. When the amygdala detects danger, it sends signals to the rest of the body to prepare for action. This preparation includes an increase in heart rate, breathing, and blood pressure, while some functions, like those in the digestive system, slow down to preserve energy. Fear is powerful because it is programmed into our nervous system.

Why would seeing a tiger in the wild cause a different response to seeing a tiger in a zoo? This is because the hippocampus, the information-processing part of the brain, reassures the amygdala what is a real threat and what is only a perceived threat.

But fear goes beyond imminent danger. Fear can also be caused by things that make us feel unsafe or unsure, such as when someone leaves us. In turn, these fears can lead to avoidance and the development of toxic behaviors, like leaving conflicts unresolved. Avoiding the source of fear doesn't cause it to go away. Instead, it can only reinforce it and make it stronger.

BEHIND THE MASK

Considering everybody's past is different, which means everyone's perspective is different, it would be wrong to assume that everybody's fears are the same.

A practical exercise would be to go through typical causes of fear and rate on a scale of 1 to 5 how relevant each fear is, with 1 being not at all and 5 causing a physical response such as anxiety and increased heart rate.

Fear of Abandonment

Growing up in a home where there is little or no emotional and physical care can wreak havoc on an adult's self-esteem. Though this might imply that a child may have lost a parent through death or divorce, it also applies to those who were absent because of long hours at work or other responsibilities despite doing the best they could.

As an adult, you may not realize that you felt neglected or abandoned during your childhood, but these experiences can still cause you to feel as if you aren't good enough as an adult and push those close to you away.

It's easier not to let anyone close than to risk the fear of being abandoned. Naturally, rejection of any kind can increase fear of abandonment.

Fear of Being Ordinary

A narcissistic trait is to feel special and superior. They are above having flaws, being weak, or making mistakes. Feelings of loneliness, self-doubt, and looking bad are for the ordinary. Your fear of being ordinary may not be as extreme, but it's still possible that perfectionism causes you to feel terrified of being anything but amazing. The fear of being ordinary can also relate to the need for important positions, power, and extreme competitiveness.

Fear of Commitment

Commitment in a relationship requires letting your guard down and letting others see that you have faults and imperfections that may even be embarrassing. There is a phenomenon called sexual narcissism, where a person creates an unrealistic image in their head by believing they are better at sex than they actually are. The fear is that a long-term relationship will expose the truth about their abilities. In some cases, commitment can feel like a loss of freedom, which can prevent you from acting on your impulses.

Fear of Insults

With an already fragile self-esteem, any insult you receive can be a crushing blow that you hold onto for much longer than usual. In some cases, people never get over a particular insult, which can exasperate the fear of receiving more. This fear can even lead to paranoia, for example, when a person makes an innocent comment, but you take it as an insult. The same applies to criticism.

Fear of Having Lies Uncovered

Imagine lies, even small exaggerations of the truth as building blocks, each one adding to the next. Remove one block and the whole structure could come crashing down. It's the same principle as lies. A lie uncovered can bring immense amounts of shame and reveal that you aren't as good as people assumed you were. In this world of lies, you are the focus of attention and admiration, and it's scary that others may find out that it's fake. They may also be paranoid about someone revealing the truth.

Fear of Remorse

Experiencing remorse can be a challenge, and the fear might be more related to remorse for a costly mistake you made rather than the hurt caused to others. Remorse might be seen as an emotional weakness or vulnerability, as it means admitting to making a mistake, which damages pride. For some, apologizing can be fearful because it can feel like the ego is threatened by admitting you have done something bad.

Fear of Gratitude

At the other end of fear of remorse, a fear of gratitude can feel like admitting help is needed. Gratitude can feel like a weakness because, in the act of needing someone, you have handed over your power. When someone does something of value or that we need, it can remove the sense of being all-powerful. Gratitude is the act of expressing appreciation for what you have, and sometimes, this can cause a fear of being judged for what you are grateful for.

Fear of the Loss of a Partner's Admiration

In many ways, the fear of losing a partner's admiration is related to previous fears. When someone you love stops admiring you, it can cause feelings of abandonment and make you realize that you aren't the most special person in a relationship and that you are ordinary.

This fear can lead to toxic behaviors such as trying to win back their love through love bombing or grand gestures.

Fear of Being Laughed at

Gelotophobia is the official name for fear of being laughed at or mocked and involves misinterpreting someone's laughter as malicious and feeling like the target of a joke.

This fear can make you feel ridiculed and lead to not trusting others and even social withdrawal. In relationships, it can cause avoidance of intimacy. This fear tends to be more common with people who have covert narcissistic traits.

Fear of Failure

Everyone, to some extent, has a fear of failure, and it goes back to the fact that it's hard to accept that we are flawed human beings. The problem for those who are struggling with toxic behaviors is that the fear of failure can be taken out on others. In such situations, they may blame those around them who don't deserve it. Additionally, they may also blame others for their lack of success.

Fear of Loss of Control

For a narcissist, a loss of control can be feared because it will expose their weaknesses, but even for those without NPD, not being in control can be terrifying because it leaves you open to negative consequences. In most cases, this will be a form of coping mechanism or defense mechanism stemming from your past. Although maintaining control can help you feel calm, it can be suffocating for those around you.

Take this opportunity to consider anything and everything that sparks fear in you. It doesn't necessarily have to be on the list above. You may fear the future or fear your own emotions. Apart from asking yourself what fears you have right now, use your journal or at least think about the following questions to know your fears better.

• Why do you fear what you fear?

• Is your fear valid, or could negative thinking get in the way?

• Are you afraid of the process or the result?

• Are you trying to protect yourself from a certain outcome?

• Have you adopted someone else's fear as your own?

• Are you scared because feelings are overwhelming?

• Do you fear uncertainty or not knowing what could happen?

Until you can accurately pinpoint your fear, you won't be able to take the steps to overcome it. Don't feel rushed to answer the questions, and know that although exploring fears can be uncomfortable, you are safe!

STARING DOWN THE FEAR

We know that avoiding fears may only fuel them and make them stronger, but at the same time, it's not as simple as just facing your fears. Before beginning any technique to overcome fears, it's essential to have the right frame of mind, and for this, you need to have some coping mechanisms prepared.

Imagine you are faced with a fear, and your body starts to react as your mind races. If you continue to stare down at the fear, the response is going to get stronger until full-blown panic kicks in. The first thing to do is gain control of the physical response by taking some time out. Try doing another activity, such as deep breathing, making your favorite drink, or walking around the block. Some people benefit from a calming playlist, which doesn't have to be slow music but any songs that put your mind in a good place.

Visualization is a great technique for putting you in the right, calm mindset for facing fears. Find a quiet, comfortable place, take a few deep breaths, and close your eyes. Picture a scene where you feel most at peace. This could be in the mountains, on a deserted beach, or by a trickling river running through a forest. Immerse yourself fully in this scene, using all your senses.

When you are ready, imagine your fear next to you in this calm place. Don't react to it. Just allow it to be present with you while you focus on your breathing and your senses. Now it's time to flip the switch! Each time you have previously pictured your fear, you will have come up with the worst possible outcome. As you remain in your calm place, imagine you have all the tools and skills necessary for a positive outcome. Create a vivid image of this positive outcome!

Susan feared talking to her parents about her personal life because the conversations usually ended up with her parents reminding her that she wasn't getting any younger and it was time to sort her life out. This resulted in Susan lying to her parents about a perfect relationship and a perfect career. During her visualization, Susan pictured herself in her parents' kitchen, where she had many fond memories of growing up. She pictured her parents sitting across from her as they sliced the fresh banana bread from the oven. She explained that her life wasn't perfect, but she was okay with that, and instead of pressuring her into taking actions that she wasn't ready for, they could support her and her decisions.

Visualization has been proven to help anxiety and can help reprogram the brain to reduce the response to fear. Remember, the more you practice, the stronger the neuro-connection becomes!

Now that your mind and body are calm, it's time to take the first step to overcoming fear.

GRADUAL EXPOSURE

If you are petrified of snakes, the last thing you want to do is visualize handling one and then allow someone to wrap a 6-foot python around you! Gradual exposure breaks down a fear and enables you to take small, manageable steps to overcome it.

Gradual exposure or exposure-based interventions is a core concept of cognitive behavioral therapy (CBT) and is typically carried out in one of four ways: in-vivo, imaginal, virtual reality, and interoceptive. In-vivo exposure involves real-life confrontation of fears. Imaginal exposure uses a person's imagination or narrative, such as a written description. This type of exposure is generally used when in-vivo exposure isn't possible, for example, past traumas or feared disasters that are unlikely. Virtual reality exposure relies on technology and is often used when real-life situations are difficult to create. Finally, interoceptive exposure focuses on triggering the physical response to fear so you learn that discomfort does not cause any harm.

It's possible to practice gradual exposure by yourself, but if you notice that you experience extreme anxiety or panic, it might be a good idea to enlist some support, whether that's a professional or someone you trust.

Let's break gradual exposure down into steps!

Step #1: Create a list of your fears

You are a step ahead because previously, we looked at potential types of fears and questions to uncover your fears. It's advisable to write down all of your fears and use this list as a brainstorming session to ensure the list is complete. Missing a fear may hinder the next steps. It may also help to group certain fears together. You may have particular emotional fears and, at the same time, a fear of spiders and dogs. Fears related to animals can be grouped together. Grouping fears is especially useful if you have many fears.

Step #2: Turn your list into a fear ladder

Use a scale of 1 to 5 to rank your levels of fear, with 0 being slight anxiety and 5 being complete panic. Next, organize these fears into a ladder where the first rung represents your least terrifying fear, while the biggest fear is placed on the top rung. Once your fears are visually organized, take the first fear on the ladder and use it to create a new ladder. For each rung on the new ladder, create steps to overcoming the fear, so every rung will be a mini-goal toward overcoming the fear. To keep the steps specific, include how long you will attempt each step, the environment you will be in, and who will be there.

Step #3: Face the first fear on the ladder

Be sure to plan your exposure to fear in advance. Know exactly what to expect and when so that you have a sense of control over the situation. Don't feel the need to rush the process, and be patient with yourself.

Face the first fear on your ladder and rate the level of anxiety or fear response. Remain with your fear until you are no longer anxious. This might mean fears that are short in duration and can be repeated multiple times so that you confront them several times. As your body adjusts to the fear, each time you repeat the first rung, your mind starts to fear it less. Keep repeating the same fear, noticing how the fear response diminishes each time. When you can face this fear, and there is no reaction, you are ready to move on to the next fear on the ladder.

Step #4: Keep practicing

Practice the steps to your fears regularly. The more often you practice, the faster you will get over them. Even once you reach the biggest of your fears and there is no longer a response, it's essential to keep practicing so that fears don't come back. If you notice this starts to happen, don't be too hard on yourself. For example, in times of stress, it may feel like you are taking one step forward and two steps back. Frequent practice will help you stay on track. Also, monitor your progress so that you can see how far you have come.

Step #5: Reward your progress

Just like any goal, every mini-goal in the process should be celebrated. Rewards should be relative to the progress made, with larger rewards given for overcoming the main fear. That's not to say that overcoming those smaller fears along the way shouldn't also be celebrated.

Step #6: Reassess your fears

As time passes, some of your fears may evolve. Some may disappear, and others may appear. The severity of fears may also change. Take your original fear ladders and reorganize them based on new levels of anxiety or fear response. If you have successfully conquered some of your fears, keep a separate list to remind you that you still need to confront them…

Tanis was terrified of showing her vulnerability and was scared that anyone who knew her weaknesses and fears would have too much power over her. Those close to her knew the bare minimum about her life, and her social withdrawal got to the point where she lacked the confidence to even say hello to people she didn't know. The first rung of her ladder was to make eye contact and say hello to her regular bus driver. The next was to talk to a friend about her day. After getting comfortable with this, her next challenge was to speak to her sister about some of the problems in her life. Finally, she was able to open up to her partner about her fear of being vulnerable.

Chris's fear of losing control caused him to micromanage every aspect of his relationship to the point where his partner was ready to leave. As two perfectly capable adults, she felt it was only fair that decisions in the home were for both of them to make. Though this may not sound like much to others, Chris began by letting his partner plan meals. It took a few weeks for him to get comfortable with this and not interfere. He then moved on to allowing his coworkers to handle more responsibility in the office. After time for reflection, Chris grew to understand that it wasn't necessarily a fear of losing control but a fear of losing financial stability that was causing his toxic behavior, so his final stage of the ladder was to hand the household budget over to his partner, which, with time and practice, he was able to do.

COGNITIVE RESTRUCTURING

There is no question that our thoughts can contribute to fears, especially negative or automatic thoughts. One thought can cause an emotion, and this emotion determines our behavior. In many cases, this is extremely useful. For example, we have a thought in the form of a goal, and this causes excitement, which, in turn, motivates our actions. However, when the thought is an irrational belief, where many fears stem from, it's necessary to work on these negative thoughts so that emotions and behaviors don't spiral out of control.

Automatic negative thoughts (or irrational beliefs) are also known as cognitive distortions. Cognitive distortions can apply to all areas of negative thinking patterns, but one that is particularly relevant is catastrophizing. Imagine your biggest fear is being laughed at while giving a presentation to coworkers. The cognitive distortion of catastrophizing means you think the situation will be far worse than it really is. Your coworkers will laugh at you, at the way you look, and at your ideas. Because of this, your project won't go through. As a result, your boss is angry, and you end up losing your job and becoming a failure. The reality is that your coworkers may have no reason to laugh at you and may actually find you amusing and be laughing with you rather than at you.

While catastrophizing and other cognitive disorders aren't recognized as mental health conditions, they can be symptoms of anxiety and depression. So, it's important to get this unhelpful thought pattern under control. This can be achieved through cognitive restructuring, another component of CBT, and other forms of talk therapy.

Use the following steps to learn how to reframe thoughts about your fears. You can also use the same structure to reframe any negative thoughts about toxic traits you may possess.

Step #1: Identify the situation

Take a moment to understand exactly what was happening that caused your negative thoughts. What happened leading up to the thought, and what were the triggers? How did this situation make you feel? Be sure to accurately identify your emotions at the time. It's easy to say, "I feel angry," and this is probably true, but would the words frustrated, humiliated, or furious be more accurate?

Step #2: Pinpoint your automatic thoughts

Automatic thoughts are those that pop into your head regularly, and you may not even realize you have them. Common automatic thoughts include:

• Nobody likes me

- Today is going to be awful

- It's all my fault

- I will never be good enough

- I shouldn't have done that

- It's all too much for me

With these examples, you can spot words associated with catastrophizing, such as nobody, all, and never. If one person doesn't like you, it doesn't mean everybody dislikes you!

Step #3: Look for evidence to support your automatic thought

Using the examples given earlier, cognitive restructuring isn't about blocking out the things we don't want to acknowledge. It's about reframing a thought so that it's based on the truth and more constructive. If you are constantly telling yourself that it's all your fault, where is the evidence? It's more likely that X was your fault, but Y wasn't.

Step #4: Look for evidence that doesn't support your automatic thought

A classic example here is when we tell ourselves we are stupid. Again, it's very possible that there was something that we shouldn't have done, and you could even go as far as saying it was a stupid thing to do. However, we are only human, and it's okay to make mistakes. This doesn't make us stupid. On the contrary, you could have a long list of qualifications, run a successful business, or have a set of skills that allows you to save lives…any of which confirms that you are not stupid.

Step #5: Rephrase your automatic thought for a balanced outlook

Based on the evidence you collected, you can now rephrase the automatic thought so that you aren't denying the truth but are representing it more accurately. For example:

• I made a mistake, but it's not the end of the world, and I can learn from it.

• What I said was accurate, but it's true I could have said it in a better way and an apology is warranted.

• Right now, my thoughts and fears are getting the better of me, but this isn't permanent. With practice, I will improve.

Robert was terrified to receive any form of criticism at work. Even the slightest feedback would be taken personally, and he knew that not only was his reaction impacting his mental health, but it was also affecting his relationships in the office. After cognitive restructuring, Robert understood that feedback wasn't a personal attack but actually, people who were trying to support him with his personal and professional growth. From here, he was able to remind himself that feedback was about his actions and not his character.

Because these types are so automatic, you need to make a conscious effort to work through the steps. Knowing that thoughts can be changed (and neuroplasticity will help this process) won't automatically change a habit you have probably had for years. I understand it's not always practical to drop everything you are doing to consider each step in detail but commit to going back to the thought when you have time.

MINDFULNESS AND MEDITATION TO CONFRONT FEARS

To understand how mindfulness and meditation can aid in overcoming fears, you should first consider how they help in dealing with stress. Right now, at this very moment, what is causing you to feel stressed?

It's almost guaranteed that any stress you are experiencing is due to something that has happened in the past or something you are worried about in the future. Fears are the same because, in this present moment, there is nothing to fear.

Learning how to spend more time in the present with mindfulness and meditation can help overcome fears as well as manage stress and anxiety. This is because they both help to calm the mind and emotions. It's excellent practice for self-control, and with a greater awareness of what is happening, it becomes easier to see reality more clearly.

Mindful meditation can be used as a way of exposure therapy when using your imagination for fears. Find a quiet, comfortable position and close your eyes. Begin by taking a few deep breaths, making sure your exhale is longer than the inhale, as this promotes more calm.

Once you feel the tension leave your body, picture your fear. If it gets too much at any time, go back to focusing on your breathing and revisit the fear once you are calm again.

Break your fear into smaller pieces and ask yourself if the fear is related to a past experience and what the likelihood is of the same thing happening again, knowing that you are now wiser than you were in the past. Is your fear about a future event, and which aspects can you control?

Pay attention to how the fear feels in your body. Are there moments when the physical sensations are more intense? If you redirect your attention to your breathing, can you control the intensity of these sensations?

Tom started practicing mindful meditation when his fear of being ordinary led to his competitiveness becoming aggressive. Though observing his fears without judgment was hard for him, he soon found inner peace and greater self-acceptance.

He discovered that his constant need for attention wasn't necessary because his worth wasn't based on standing out from or being better than others.

Mindful meditation isn't easy, especially if the practice is new to you. When I began, I could only last a couple of minutes before my mind began to wander. Guided meditations are incredibly helpful in getting you started.

Using a video or script gives your mind a voice and instructions to follow rather than attempting to do it alone. There are plenty of videos online, but here are some of my favorites that have helped me in the past.

**Guided Mindfulness Meditation
on Overcoming Anxiety**

Starting with shorter guided meditation videos and working your way up to the longer ones can be beneficial. Even five minutes can have a big impact on your mental well-being.

**LET GO of Anxiety, Fear &
Worries Meditation**

JOURNALING TO SELF-REFLECT ON FEARS

Journaling is rather underrated, considering the numerous proven benefits.

Research has shown that journaling can have a positive effect on anxiety, depression, and recovery from emotional trauma and that there is an even greater improvement when journaling for more than 30 days (Sohal et al., 2022).

The key to effective journaling is consistency rather than length or frequency. You may prefer to write for ten minutes daily, or you may be happier when you spend 30 minutes writing once a week. To be consistent, you should set an alarm on your phone because we all know how hectic life can get.

Journaling doesn't have to involve a traditional notebook and pen. You can use a document on your computer or phone, or you can even use voice notes to record how you process your fears and emotions. You may find that writing comes easily to you, but if you struggle to get started, these journal prompts can help.

• Complete the sentence. I'm afraid of _____ But my biggest fear is _____

• When did your fears begin?

• What does facing your fears mean to you?

• What is the worst-case scenario that could realistically happen??

- Personify your fear. If my fear were a person, it would
  _____

- Continue to imagine your fear as a person. Ask your fear what it hopes to achieve in your life.

- What do you need to overcome your fear?

- How is your fear limiting your life?

- What healthy steps can you take to overcome your fear?

- How would your future self handle this fear?

- What does your life look like once your fears are behind you?

Lily feared relationships, being judged, rejected, and failing as a partner. Though both parents had been happily remarried for well over 20 years, it wasn't until Lily started journaling that she could trace her fears back to their divorce, which happened almost 30 years ago when she was still a young child. Despite hardly remembering the divorce, Lily traced her own fear of failure back to her parents' failed relationship, and with this realization, she was better able to process her past and present emotions.

Facing fears can be a little bit like the darkness before the light, the dip of a rollercoaster before the high. You have to courageously work through the hard stuff in order to see brighter results. It's this light at the end of the tunnel that will help you in the next chapter of your life, giving you a fresh start in your relationships and making your communication and connections more positive!

CHAPTER FIVE: A NEW LEAF

> *Effective communication is 20% what you know and 80% how you feel about what you know.*
>
> *JIM ROHN*

In all my years as a life coach, this is one of the quotes that rings so true to me and many clients. Communication is a tricky thing, and one of the biggest assumptions we make is that communication is complete once the words have been spoken.

Whether it's how you feel about what you know or what you think you know, this 80 percent has a massive impact on the other person's response. The cycle continues when you listen and only hear what you want to hear. Imagine if your first sentence was only 20 percent effective and the second was even less so. As a result, communication quickly breaks down.

The L in the REFLECT framework is all about learning healthy patterns of interactions, but before we begin, it's crucial to put past communications behind us. We will start by looking at what often goes wrong in our communication, but this isn't a chance to revisit the past and beat yourself up about how you may have mishandled situations. These past mistakes are now learning opportunities!

TURNING THE TIDE

Poor communication in a toxic relationship of any kind is a huge stressor for both parties. No relationship is problem-free, but in a toxic one, poor communication means problems aren't resolved quickly or easily; in fact, it's more likely that they escalate. In the next chapter, we will take time to consider how others feel. For now, think about the last time you fell into one of the following negative communication patterns or were on the receiving end and how you felt.

Complaints and Criticism

During the "honeymoon" phase of a relationship, the other person is flawless, but then, like yourself, imperfections become apparent, and the criticism begins. A person can quickly start to feel like nothing they do is good enough when complaints and criticism become the norm.

In fact, criticism is one of the Four Horsemen, which are four behaviors that are a strong sign of a relationship failure. Don't forget that a complaint addresses a behavior, while criticism attacks a person's character.

Imagine a person who spends all morning cleaning their house (on top of their own work) only for their partner to come home and complain right away that the garden is a mess.

It's not a criticism, but it still leaves the other person questioning why they bother.

Contempt

Contempt is a form of mean and nasty behavior that goes beyond criticism. It's another of the Four Horsemen that can be displayed through words of disrespect, mocking, sarcasm, and name-calling. It can also be shown in negative body language, such as eye scrolling, hand gestures, scoffing, or huffing in response.

This behavior is a direct attack on a person's self-esteem and is fueled by deep negative thoughts about the other person.

Contempt can also be displayed as hostile humor, something that Freud called "disguised aggression."

For some, it could look like a person is being funny, but really, their humor is only intended to cause psychological pain.

An example would be someone saying to their coworker, "If you think someone is laughing at you, they probably are." It doesn't sound like much, but it can cause the receivers to doubt themselves in all interactions.

Defensiveness

The third of the Four Horsemen is often a response to criticism. Someone who feels under attack may become defensive as a way of self-protection. However, it's often just a sign of shifting responsibility by blaming others and making excuses. When responsibility isn't taken, it's easy to fall into the victim mentality trap.

Picture a couple discussing their finances, and one mentions how the other spent $100 over the budget. Defensiveness would reply, "Well, last month, you spent $150 over the budget." It doesn't solve anything; it's just an attempt to excuse the mistake.

Stonewalling

If you have teens, you may well have come up against stonewalling, but this is due to their age and developmental stages rather than a sign of toxic behavior. Stonewalling, the last of the Four Horsemen is when a person tries to communicate an issue with you, but instead of responding effectively, you go silent, respond with monosyllabic answers (much like teens), change the subject, or act busy. In some cases, this can be a self-soothing response or a chance to calm down, but it's an evasive tactic that prevents you from dealing with the problem at hand. It can come across as if you don't care about the situation or the person trying to talk to you.

A common example of stonewalling nowadays is picking up and using your phone when someone is trying to have a serious conversation with you. There is nothing on your phone that is more important than the conversation at hand.

Gaslighting

Gaslighting is high up on the list of negative communication patterns and a narcissistic form of manipulation. This is a type of psychological control where misleading and untrue information is fed to a victim in order to have them question their own version of events, their reality, and, in extreme cases, their sanity. While questioning their own self-identity and self-worth, the gaslighter is able to emotionally, physically, or financially control the person. Gaslighting often starts with subtle acts of manipulation, sometimes even in the early stages of a relationship.

If a person tries to explain that they are feeling controlled in a relationship and expresses this, the gaslighter may respond with, "Are you sure I am trying to control you?" sparking the seeds of doubt. They would follow up their question with a justification that comes across as caring, such as "I'm only trying to help you make the best choices."

Steamrolling and Interrupting

In some ways, steamrolling and interrupting can be related to stonewalling and defensive communication, as they are techniques that result in a person not being able to express themselves. Steamrolling involves talking over a person or quickly changing the subject, and of course, interrupting someone means that they don't have a chance to finish what they are saying, whether that's their thoughts or feelings. Both steamrolling and interrupting can be incredibly frustrating and lead to arguments.

A father repeatedly interrupts his young daughter, which frustrates her. Due to her age, she is unable to control her emotions, so the two end up shouting at each other. This pattern of negativity is only made worse when the daughter, who learned from a poor example, interrupts her father, and things escalate.

Negative Interpretations

Negative interpretations go back to making inaccurate assumptions. We hear what a person has said, though perhaps not the correct message. Then, in our minds, we rewrite the message. Sometimes, we will rewrite this narrative to make it fit with our own thoughts or beliefs. There are two ways this can backfire. It's possible that you hear something and misinterpret it as an insult. Or you hear what is meant to be constructive criticism and catastrophize it so that it becomes more of a big deal than it ever was. With today's digital communication and, in particular, emojis, we have to be careful not to negatively interpret written messages.

Imagine a parent who has asked a favor from their adult child but they can't do it. After half an hour of sending the message but not receiving a response, the parent texts back, "Don't worry, your brother will do it when he comes for lunch on Sunday." This could be a genuine message not to cause stress, but it could also be interpreted negatively as if the brother is the golden child who comes home for lunch every week and fixes all the problems.

Aggressive or Threatening Communication

Unfortunately, the list of potential aggressive or threatening communication is extensive and can be subjective, especially among different cultures. Some cultures naturally speak louder than others, which can be perceived as aggressive by those from different cultures. Some American cultures (indigenous, Alaskan native, and Latin American) tend to speak with a softer tone than, for example, certain Eastern Asian cultures. Additionally, for some Asian cultures, direct eye contact may be considered aggressive (Think Culture Health, n. d.).

Overall, aggressive and threatening communication is any form of communication in which the other person feels disregarded, disrespected, or victimized. The person will try to dominate a situation, be loud to the point of overbearing, and have low levels of tolerance and plenty of criticism and interruptions.

Passive-Aggressive Messages

Though a person may not feel as threatened as with aggressive communication, that doesn't mean passive-aggressive communication isn't just as upsetting. A passive-aggressive communicator will often agree with what a person says but then "forget" what it was or not do what was asked of them because they "forgot." Procrastination and backhanded compliments can be a form of passive-aggressive. If passive-aggressive communicators have manipulative tendencies, they may also use gaslighting to make the other person question what they really meant.

One woman walks into her friend's house and says, "I wish I could be the type of person who could cope with all this clutter." Although it may come across as a compliment, in reality, they are just insulting the other person's home.

The situation would be even worse if the woman added a follow-up comment along the lines of "Oh, you know I didn't mean it like that, silly."

With these negative communication patterns in mind, there is one particular word I would like you to focus on —patterns! I would be lying if I said that my wife and I never raised our voices, and you would be hard-pressed to find a parent who has never complained about their children!

These patterns become problematic when they are frequent and cause significant damage to your communication and relationships.

Now that you have identified your own negative patterns, the only way to truly turn the tide is by recognizing your mistakes.

THE POWER OF AN APOLOGY

Apologizing is hard at the best of times, but it is a crucial step in mending broken connections. Whether a person chooses to forgive you or not is up to them, but you can greatly increase the possibility with a genuine apology.

Apologizing gives you a chance to be humble and honest, as well as taking accountability for your actions. For the other person, it's a way for them to find their dignity after you have hurt them. For both of you, it's a chance to repair a damaged relationship.

A genuine apology has four elements:

• Taking responsibility for the offense and admiting that this behavior isn't acceptable.

• An explanation for what happened without making excuses.

• To express your remorse, to let others know you regret it, or that you are ashamed, even humiliated by your actions.

• To make amends, whether that is rectifying a wrong in the cause of physical damage or committing to being more sensitive to the emotional suffering caused.

Look at the difference between the two apologies:

1. "Sorry for whatever happened; mistakes were made."

2. "I'm sorry for losing my temper. I had ´a hard day, which I know isn't an excuse because you have had a hard day, too. I promise to try and express myself better next time."

Not only is the second sentence specific, but the use of "I" in the beginning shows how the person is taking responsibility for the mistake. In contrast, the first sentence uses the passive voice, which avoids accountability and does not specify who made the mistake.

This art of a genuine apology takes practice, and it may help to write your thoughts down and read them to the person rather than send a message or email. It's true that a message or email is better than nothing, but face-to-face will deliver a more heartfelt apology.

BUILDING BRIDGES, NOT WALLS

An apology is a good start to breaking down the walls you have built between yourself and others, but in order to build a bridge, it's essential to make changes in the way you communicate. In the 1960s, clinical psychologist Marshall Rosenberg developed nonviolent communication as a solution to address the violence in his hometown. Today, nonviolent communication (NVC) is a strategy to help improve communication in all types of relationships, but it is particularly effective in romantic relationships.

Essentially, NVC is the use of compassionate language and has several benefits. NVC helps build self-awareness as you start to pay more attention to your feelings and needs. Honesty increases as you get better at communicating those needs, which can lead to greater intimacy and compassion for yourself and others. As you get better at responding rather than reacting, relationships experience fewer conflicts.

To turn negative communication patterns into nonviolent

communication, it's worth examining how past habits can be transformed into the core elements of NVC:

- Evaluations become observations

- Thoughts become emotions

- Strategies become universal needs

- Demands become requests

Let's explore these concepts in more detail.

Observations

Observations refer to raw information that we directly hear or see. This sounds simple enough, but the brain has a habit of taking an observation and turning it into a story, which then transforms into an evaluation. If somebody arrives late, your observation would be that they arrived late. However, if you say they are always late, it becomes an evaluation because you have mixed the observation with a generalization and an attack on the person.

Observations are wonderful because, as the first stage of communication, they increase the chances of the other person listening to you because your words aren't just another criticism. In return, they will be more willing to respond to you in a compassionate way rather than reacting to your words. These observations also reduce the use of right or wrong thinking, which tends to happen in evaluations, and enable you to use accountable language.

Nevertheless, it's not easy to separate observations from evaluations. You need to practice leaving judgments and interpretations out of the message. To get better at this, treat your observations as snapshots from a video recorder. A video recorder can only capture what you can see and hear!

Emotions

It's scary to open up about our feelings, but considering people aren't mind readers, difficult conversations need an emotional explanation. As soon as you tell someone that you are anxious, hurt, or experiencing any other emotion, the other person can start to understand your needs without making assumptions. Expressing how you feel also allows you to take responsibility for your own emotions rather than coming across as blaming others.

Expressing our emotions can have two potential problems. The first is that emotions can often come across as thoughts. The second is that, if not expressed correctly, it can seem that you are making others responsible for how you feel.

If you say to someone, "I feel that you are making fun of this situation," although you have the word "feel," it's a thought you are having because you aren't defining exactly how you feel. In the second scenario, notice the difference between saying, "You make me feel angry when you don't listen" and "I feel angry when you don't listen," In the first sentence, even though the word "feel" is used, the other person is the source of your anger, whereas in the second sentence, you are owning your emotion.

Needs

All humans have a basic set of needs, such as food, water, shelter, rest, and connection. When these needs aren't met, our survival is threatened. NVC doesn't just take into account the basic needs but also considers our core values and deepest desires. These will look different for each individual, but common needs can include collaboration, support, respect, consistency, and understanding.

The key to expressing needs is to keep the need universal. This way, the other person doesn't feel like an unmet need is a criticism or a failure of theirs.

If you were to say, "I need support," you would be expressing a universal need. However, as soon as you say, "I need support from you," you would be implying they don't give you support.

From the previous example, you can see that the words "I need" don't automatically indicate a universal need that increases connections. I could tell you right now that I need a cold drink while lying by a pool. This describes a strategy to achieve the basic human needs (hydration and rest). Again, avoid strategies in your messages.

If you were talking to your teen, instead of saying, "I need you to text me every hour," which sounds controlling, you can say, "I need reassurance you are safe."

Requests

For needs to be met and willingly, we need to ensure our requests are clear and reasonable. It's important to remember that other people cannot read our minds. If your request isn't specific enough, it's likely that your needs won't be met, and the other person may become frustrated due to the lack of clarity. For instance, asking someone to be more considerate doesn't provide enough direction, but asking them to consider the feelings of others during a meeting provides precise direction.

To reduce conflict, it's also critical that requests don't come across as complaints. Even if you follow the first steps and say, "I feel like you never have time for me," it still comes across as negative compared with asking, "Could we make plans for the weekend so that we can spend some quality time together?"

Don't forget that everybody has the right to decline a request, even if you have expressed your request in the best way possible. To prevent any conflicts from arising, approach the situation with curiosity. Without being defensive, demanding, or complaining, ask why they said no and if there is anything you can do to help.

To master the skill of nonviolent communication, practice with the following sentence:

When _____ (your observation), I feel_____ (your emotion) because I need _____ (universal need). Would you be able to _____ (your request)?

Here are some examples:

When *I see dirty clothes all over the floor*, I feel *frustrated because* I need t*o feel like more than just the maid*. In the future, would you please be able to *put your laundry in the basket?*

When *I sent you the messages, and you didn't reply*, I felt *worried that* something had happened to you, and I needed *to know you were safe*. In the future, *can you reply, even if it's just a short message?*

When *I sense that you aren't listening to me*, I feel *ignored,* and I need *to know that my opinions are valued too*. Next time we have a serious conversation, *could you consider leaving your phone somewhere else?*

Ideally, you want to keep your sentences below 45 to 50 words so it docsn't become a long-winded speech. Here are some top tips to implement NVC into your communications:

• Actively listen to what other people are telling you. I know there is a lot of thought and concentration going on, but if you don't listen to the actual message someone gives you, your next observation will be inaccurate.

• Take a breath before you respond, and if that's not enough, kindly ask the person if you can have a minute or two. Calm yourself, and then go back to the conversation. There is no pressure to respond at the moment!

• Make sure the other person is comfortable talking to you about their feelings. If bridges have been burned, it may take time for them to speak openly to you. Pushing them or resorting to manipulation is crossing their boundaries.

• Accept that some people will not care about your feelings. Remember that you are only responsible for your thoughts, feelings, and actions.

• Practice compassion. Recognize the efforts you have taken to implement NVC, knowing that it wasn't easy. Be kind to yourself when you don't get it right the first time. It's a process!

NVC can actually be used by abusers as a form of manipulation. In the final section, we will discover how to rid your words and actions of manipulative traits.

BREAK FREE FROM MANIPULATIVE WORDS AND ACTIONS

Not all manipulation is obvious. If this is something you have been doing for a long time, it has become second nature, and you may not even consider it manipulative behavior. Manipulation is any use of emotional pressure to control another person's decisions or actions. Here are some ways you could be manipulating others, intentionally or unintentionally:

• You use guilt trips to get what you want

• You are determined to get your own way, even taking advantage of the kindness of others

- You are nice to people you don't like because you will gain from it

- You throw around threats and promises like they are going out of style, all to bend others to your will

- You make some empty threats and promises to get your way

- When someone says no, you see this as an opportunity to continue persuading that person

- You disrespect people's refusal and will resort to other tactics to change their mind

- You criticize other people's friends and family in order to create distance between them

- You withhold attention and/or affection until someone does what you want

- You have issues with jealousy

- You tend to create drama for your benefit, so much so you could have your own drama show

Not all manipulation is bad. When you smile at another person, your intention is to encourage them to smile, which is still manipulating their emotions. But when this turns into coercion, manipulation can have extremely harmful effects on relationships. Other people will be full of negative thoughts about you that can lead to perceived negative emotions. As awful as it is to hear, some people may dread being around you because of the effect you have on how they feel. Your manipulation can cause others to doubt their reality.

Self-Esteem

As the motivation for manipulation is power and control, it's essential to start by improving your self-esteem to overcome your insecurities. This can be done by journaling your achievements and using positive affirmations. There is nothing like comparing yourself to others to bring down your self-esteem. Instead, remind yourself that self-worth isn't based on tangible items, status, or wealth. Even with your flaws, you are good enough as a human being—that's self-worth!

Triggers

While working on your self-esteem, take the time to recognize patterns in your manipulative behavior. Noticing what triggers your manipulative traits through awareness and reflection will help you identify causes to stop the behavior before it happens. It will help if you ask those closest to you for some feedback, especially if you struggle to spot such behaviors. Ask them how your manipulative behaviors made them feel in the past.

Asserting Yourself

You want to avoid passive-aggressive and aggressive communication and master the skills of assertive communication. To do this, remember the HONEST acronym:

• **H:** Hold your ground. Maintain your position and beliefs respectfully, but know that you aren't always right

• **O:** Open-mindedness. Actively listen to others and consider their perspectives without judgment

- **N:** Nonverbal cues. Be aware of your tone of voice, especially for sarcasm. Check that facial expressions, hand movements, and posture are not overbearing or threatening

- **E:** Express yourself clearly. Be honest, direct, and concise when expressing thoughts and emotions. Sometimes, fewer words are more effective!

- **S:** Self-awareness. Constantly be mindful of your emotions, and calm your emotions before responding

- **T:** Take responsibility. Be accountable for your words and actions. When things go wrong, admit your part in it

Respect Boundaries

When someone says "no," you accept and respect it. There are exceptions. If that person has said no, it's because they have a boundary in place that protects their emotional, physical, and mental needs.

Not everyone has healthy boundaries in place and will struggle to say no. In this case, you need to read signs of their discomfort. Do they pause before responding? Do they take a step back? Are they fidgeting?

Others will use sentences that mean no without saying the word, for example, "Thanks for the invite, but I can't make it." Just because you don't hear the word no, it doesn't mean you can attempt to change their mind.

Manipulative people tend to have weak boundaries themselves. It would be beneficial for you to work on developing healthy boundaries to see how useful they are as a form of self-protection and just what it feels like when someone crosses one of your boundaries!

There is one thing that I have said before, but I want to reiterate it. You will likely be feeling quite low about yourself after considering how your past behavior has affected the lives of others, more so if you were unaware of the extent of the impact. There are two paths ahead of you.

One will lead to negative thought patterns and potentially worse symptoms of anxiety and depression if you beat yourself up over the past. The second path leads to accepting that these mistakes were made and making sure that the techniques in this chapter are implemented and the same mistakes aren't repeated!

One negative trait we have yet to discuss is empathy, which is so important for healthy communication and building meaningful relationships that it warrants a chapter of its own.

CHAPTER SIX: HEART WIDE OPEN

> *I think we all have empathy. We may not have enough courage to display it.*

MAYA ANGELOU

One of the common things we hear about narcissists, or at least those with narcissistic personality disorder, is that they have little to no empathy. But what if we took a different perspective, much like Angelou?

What if empathy was like a seed already within you, but it just needs the right conditions to germinate and thrive? And what if, for the conditions to be achieved, you need to break down your emotional barriers and let other people in? It's only natural that this requires some courage!

WHAT EXACTLY IS EMPATHY?

Previously, we discussed the importance of perspective and seeing things from different points of view. Empathy takes this to the next level and enables you to connect on an emotional level and feel the same things they are feeling. There are three types of empathy:

- **Affective empathy:** The ability to appropriately respond to another person's emotions. For example, not reacting to anger with anger.

- **Somatic empathy:** The ability to feel what someone else is feeling. You can feel someone's frustration when they can't do something.

- **Cognitive empathy:** The ability to understand a person's emotional response to a situation. Your child is crying because they are scared of the dark, and you recognize that this must be scary for them.

Some people make the mistake of interchanging the words empathy and sympathy. The meanings are similar, but still with a significant difference.

Sympathy is understanding that someone is going through a particular experience, especially a difficult one, and feeling sorry or compassion for that person. Empathy is sharing the same emotions.

Brené Brown, a research professor whose focus is on vulnerability, shame, and empathy, explains sympathy with one clear example:

"I'm over here, and you're over there. I'm sorry for you, and I'm sad for you. And while I'm sorry that happened to you, let's be clear: I'm over here." (Abram, 2013)

For someone to have empathy, they would be standing "over there" feeling the same sadness.

At this point, it's worth noting that narcissists are often attracted to empaths; it's like the yin to their yang. Narcissists crave validation and attention. Empaths have high levels of compassion and are quick to validate the needs of a narcissist because they feel their pain.

Empathy is one of the five core elements of emotional intelligence, the others being self-awareness, self-regulation, social skills, and motivation. Self-awareness and self-regulation refer to the ability to recognize one's own emotions and manage them. Someone with toxic traits may not have problems with self-awareness and self-regulation, but tapping into another person's emotions can be exceptionally challenging—but not impossible!

THE NARCISSIST AND EMPATHY DEBATE

After telling his wife she was a hindrance and replaceable at any moment, she left him. Marcos lost everything and hit rock bottom. Throughout his life, Marcos felt that he was different from everyone else. He couldn't understand why he got so angry when he saw other people suffering. Online research informed him that therapy was the only way forward for him, which is when he was diagnosed with NPD.

His lack of empathy has been hard for him, especially raising three children. He genuinely couldn't feel the feelings they had when they were upset or needed comfort. However, thanks to therapy, he has been able to develop more cognitive empathy. Although he can't share their suffering, he has learned how to understand why they are feeling that way.

Marcos is in the minority! It is estimated that between 2 and 16 percent of people with NPD seek professional help (Ambardar & Bienenfeld, 2023). As we have seen, someone with NPD won't notice that they have a problem. Furthermore, they may even feel that their lack of empathy is a benefit for them. Not having to deal with those pesky emotions keeps them on the path to success.

Whether it's NPD or you are dealing with narcissistic traits, empathy is a complex matter. Brain scans have shown that people with NPD have less gray matter in the left anterior insula, the area of the brain related to empathy, compassion, and cognitive function, as well as abnormal levels of white matter in the anterior insula, where compassion is processed and generated (Graham, n.d.). These parts of the brain might be different from someone who doesn't have NPD, but it doesn't mean that these parts are nonexistent. Empathy is generated, just not used.

This explains why some narcissists have the ability to show immense empathy toward their pet or a small child but then appear emotionless with others. Some will have the ability to withhold empathy as a way of controlling another person, while others have the ability to show or even fake empathy, especially when they are going to gain from it.

Because the root cause of narcissistic behaviors is a severe lack of self-esteem, it's also worth considering that a lack of empathy is a form of self-protection. It's possible that some situations allow the narcissist to show their vulnerability, and other situations that make them feel helpless cause them to withhold their empathy, more so if the situation causes them to feel shame.

Further research has shown that narcissists can empathize but only when instructed to put themselves in the position of the other person. When watching a video of domestic abuse, the narcissistic participants showed similar levels of empathy to non-narcissistic participants when told to imagine how the victim felt. Those who weren't given instructions showed no empathy. In the same study, participants' heart rates (an indication of empathy) were also measured while they watched a video about a couple breaking up. Narcissists who were instructed to see the perspective of the couple had an increased heart rate compared with those who weren't given instructions (Mitrokostas, 2018).

All of this confirms that narcissists and those with NPD can develop and show empathy, but there is no guarantee that this is automatic.

WHEN IT DOESN'T COME EASY

Let's take away the idea that you are unwilling to express empathy but that it's extremely difficult for you. You may have certain barriers that make you come across as uncaring and even, on occasion, hurtful.

Cognitive Biases

Cognitive biases are inaccurate thinking patterns that impact how we see the world. A few in particular can prevent or reduce empathy.

The first is confirmation bias, which involves the habit of looking for, interpreting, and remembering information that supports or confirms our beliefs and opinions. At the same time, we ignore anything that goes against our beliefs and opinions. This could lead to showing less empathy to those who contradict you.

Fundamental attribution error is when we blame a person's behavior on their character rather than considering all contributing factors to the situation.

If your partner is at home on the sofa, you might be tempted to label them as lazy instead of considering that they are ill. Similarly, if a team member can't finish a task, you might assume they are incompetent and not because they didn't have the necessary resources.

In-group bias refers to the tendency to prefer and trust people within our own groups, whether that's friendships, religion, or workplace departments. This is particularly dangerous because there isn't just the risk of showing less or no empathy to those outside your group. There is also the risk of discrimination.

Dehumanization

With an inflated sense of self, dehumanization can be a common barrier for those with narcissistic traits. Dehumanizing a person is when we devalue a person, dismiss them, or deprive them of positive human qualities.

Making someone out to be less than human is almost the polar opposite of empathy! Aside from derogating people, it makes aggression and harming others easier.

There is an argument to be made that dehumanization is a strategy for emotional regulation.

For example, some healthcare workers may dehumanize patients as a form of self-protection from the suffering they witness daily. Nevertheless, it's important not to use this as an excuse for improper behavior or a lack of empathy.

Victim Blaming

An extreme example of this is when someone blames the victim of a crime rather than the criminal. When you hear about someone who has been raped, you question why they didn't fight or run instead of recognizing that it was unquestionably the rapist in the wrong.

You may find yourself using phrases like "If you had just answered your phone, I wouldn't have lost my temper." Although this might be true, there could have been a number of reasons why they didn't answer the phone, and your temper is your responsibility. The angry outburst pulls all the attention to your feelings and not what the other person is going through.

Lack of Self-Awareness

Emotional intelligence is fortunately a part of most school curriculums today, but for us, the closest we got to emotional intelligence was learning adjectives! This means that the majority of adults lack self-awareness. Even if you are aware of your own emotions, there is the obstacle of managing these emotions and the reactions they cause. Considering the variables involved, the bigger obstacle is understanding how your words and actions affect another person.

A simple joke can cause one person to laugh in hysterics, but the next person could find it incredibly offensive. A partner could brush off your harsh words one day, but if they have had a stressful day themselves, they can find your attitude to be frustrating or hurtful.

Fear and Insecurity

This is another barrier that can't be used as an excuse, but understanding how fear and insecurity can impact your ability to empathize with others is a great step forward. You may have many fears, but let's take the fear of abandonment as an example.

A fear of abandonment is also an insecurity. It can lead to overbearing behavior and codependency. You may go out of your way to ensure that someone doesn't leave you, taking away any independence they have. Your fears may push the other person away because it is better that they leave now than later on. Either way, you are taking away their emotions in place of your own. You aren't the only person with fears and insecurities!

Fatigue and Stress

Exhaustion can affect our ability to pay attention and actively listen to those we are communicating with. Actively listening isn't just about listening to words, but it's also about reading a person's body language to understand better how a person is feeling. It's very likely that an empath will give you a verbal message that is not necessarily true; they say what they think they want you to hear. Getting better at reading other people will allow you to see if their nonverbal cues match their verbal message. This is especially true of microexpressions, which are flashes of emotions that are harder to fake.

As for stress, it has a habit of consuming our minds and distracting us. Constant worry about what has happened and what may happen inhibits our attention too. If this is combined with cognitive biases ("They can't possibly have as much stress as I do"), you will find it hard to empathize with the problems of others.

Multitasking

Imagine the number of times you have been in the kitchen doing dishes, preparing dinner, thinking about the messages you haven't sent yet, and all the other things you attempt to juggle at once. At the same time, your loved one is telling you about your day. You don't have to be a narcissist or have toxic traits to miss out on what they are telling you. However, not giving this person the respect they deserve is a lack of respect. Somebody once told me that if your children want to tell you something, it's essential that you put aside everything else and listen because, at that moment, you are the most important person they want to talk to.

This same principle should be applied to anyone who wants or needs your attention.

At first, you may have thought that overcoming your barriers to empathy would require a huge effort. In reality, they are all small changes that only require your motivation and can make unbelievable changes in how people perceive you. Next, we will move on to these changes.

5 PRACTICAL WAYS TO STEPPING INTO SOMEONE ELSE'S SHOES

If developing empathy requires motivation, the first thing to do is understand why you want to work on this skill. Why do you need to increase your empathy? Is it to strengthen your relationship or to connect better with your children? Do you need empathy to achieve a personal or professional goal?

Your why shouldn't be based on things like wealth, popularity, or other things that narcissism encourages you to chase. Jim Carey made a great point about this:

"I think everybody should get rich and famous and do everything they ever dreamed of so they can see that it's not the answer." (Burns, 2021)

To help you consider your why, ask yourself what makes you happy. Then, ask yourself what makes you feel fulfilled. You might think they are the same, but happiness is a short-term emotion, whereas fulfillment is a long-term state of being. Receiving your paycheck will make you happy, but fulfillment comes when you take some of that paycheck and use it to help others, for example.

Paint a vivid picture of how empathy will help you in life. Imagine what it would feel like for you and your team as you hit your goals together.

At the same time, consider how your low levels of empathy are holding you back from all the things you want to achieve. When this picture is clear, you will have the motivation to start overcoming barriers.

Mastering Self-Awareness

From my perspective, self-awareness is the cornerstone of empathy and a great place to start to overcome several barriers. Self-awareness lets you focus on yourself and your actions, thoughts, and emotions. You may think that having narcissistic traits means you overly focus on yourself and should be focusing more on others, but this teaches you how to pay attention to the reality of what you do rather than an internal story that you tell yourself. It also helps with self-control, confidence, and self-esteem.

If you want to be able to understand the emotions of others, you first have to understand your own, and this requires expanding your vocabulary. In the past, my emotional vocabulary was limited to words like fine, good, stressed, or angry. But I realized that these words are not enough to describe how I am feeling accurately. So, I banned myself from using these words to describe how I was feeling and forced myself to pause throughout the day and choose one of the 27 main emotions we experience:

- Admiration
- Adoration
- Aesthetic appreciation
- Amusement
- Anxiety
- Awe
- Awkwardness
- Boredom
- Calmness
- Confusion
- Craving
- Disgust
- Empathetic pain
- Entrancement
- Envy
- Excitement
- Fear
- Horror
- Interest
- Joy

- Nostalgia
- Romance
- Sadness
- Satisfaction
- Sexual desire
- Sympathy
- Triumph

Self-aware people also take time for self-reflection, whether that's through journaling or taking time to think. They are able to recognize their strengths and areas for improvement. They have a clear idea of their values and beliefs and will make decisions that align with them. Finally, they also understand the reason behind their behaviors. Whether an action is good or bad, ask yourself why you did what you did.

How to Find Common Ground with Others

Aside from increasing empathy, common ground can bring people closer together, especially through reduced conflict. It makes forming new friendships easy and can also help to disrupt echo chambers where everyone's views are the same. Common ground isn't just about interests but also about finding topics and opinions you can agree on. It's okay if you disagree. The important thing is to accept this and try to find something you can agree on, even if it's just agreeing to disagree.

Open-ended and follow-up questions are excellent opportunities for finding common ground. Instead of asking someone, "Did you enjoy your holiday?" which will lead to a yes or no answer, ask, "What did you enjoy about your holiday?" Perhaps they tried a hobby you like or a food that you have never tried. My only advice with open-ended questions is to avoid sensitive topics that could easily lead to conflicting opinions, such as religion and politics.

Taking a genuine interest in other people provides the chance to see aspects of yourself in others, and it's this connection that makes empathy easier. Once you have started opening up more with those who make it easy to empathize, broaden your horizons, and actively seek out people who are different from you to enhance this skill.

Reading The Hidden Messages

Before trying to decode the not-so-obvious messages, life and empathy would be less challenging if you make the effort to listen actively. Actively listening means hearing what a person is saying but also tapping into their thoughts and feelings. The first step toward active listening is to give a person your full attention without tangible distractions like mobile phones or mental noise. Mental noise refers to the continuous stream of thoughts about things like what you need to add to your shopping list or what time you said you would meet your friend.

Mental noise that is particularly damaging is judgment. Instead of listening, your mind might judge what a person is wearing, why they are telling you the things they are telling you, or worse, negative thoughts like how ridiculous they sound. There is no time for judgment when you are listening, and we have already seen that multitasking doesn't work in our favor. To tame the judgments, think about how hard it was for this person to have this conversation with you, especially if you haven't been the kindest person to approach in the past.

Interrupting a person is a surefire way to quickly kill any empathy you have created. It shows a lack of respect, and it throws the other person's thought trail off. If you interrupt a person, you haven't given them a chance to finish what they were going to say, which could be exactly what you interrupt them for. Never assume you know what they are about to say, and don't start forming your response until they have finished speaking.

As for reading emotions, the eyes and mouth often give away the most information. It's best to look at images online of different facial expressions to better distinguish subtle differences. After facial expressions, the tone of voice can tell you more about a person's emotions. A tense voice can indicate anger compared with a softer tone, which may suggest that someone is feeling nervous. Sometimes, gestures are easier to read. Look for people fidgeting as a sign of anxiety or nerves, stepping away from you in order to create distance, or blocking themselves by crossing arms or placing an object between you.

It's necessary to remember that not one verbal or nonverbal cue will give you all the answers to a person's emotions. Focusing on one area won't give you the whole picture. It's best to practice scanning for all nonverbal cues while listening. It may sound like a lot to do at once, but you will get better at reading emotions with practice.

Be Curious About What's Beyond Your Comfort Zone

Imagine following the same routine every day, from talking to the same people to listening to the same news channel. Without vast exposure to the differences in the world around you, you aren't going to have the opportunity to see different perspectives, and this is a sure way to fuel your biases and stereotypes of others.

In many ways, stepping out of your comfort zone requires the same steps as overcoming fears. It's about understanding what makes you feel uncomfortable and managing the emotions that this discomfort creates. Then, you can break down the steps to what makes you feel uncomfortable into more manageable steps.

Stepping out of your comfort zone forces you to understand what it is like when other people feel confused, embarrassed, nervous, or self-conscious. Previously, you may have mocked someone for their clothing choice, making them feel self-conscious. When you actively choose to wear something that makes you feel self-conscious, you have firsthand experience of the other person's emotions.

Curiosity is a great way to break down your biases toward those who are in different groups than yourself. Take some time to learn about different cultures, traditions, and beliefs. Watch movie genres you wouldn't normally watch or books written by authors from around the world. Just as we practice looking at things from a fictional character's point of view, we can also do the same to get better at understanding and sharing their emotions.

Manage Your Distractions

A little bit of self-care goes a long way to managing exhaustion and stress. Self-care isn't about spoiling yourself or luxury. It's about taking care of your physical and emotional needs.

These simple acts put you in a better position to fulfill your responsibilities, but they also provide you with the energy for self-awareness, managing your stress, and taking care of those who need you.

Self-care is an individual practice, but self-awareness will help you tune into your needs.

There are various areas of self-care. For each of the following, think of a way that you could practice self-care that will help you develop more empathy:

- **Physical self-care:** eating a balanced diet, drinking enough water, getting regular exercise, creating a healthy sleep routine

- **Mental self-care:** setting goals, journaling, learning new skills, working on personal growth

- **Emotional self-care:** setting boundaries, journaling about your feelings, finding healthy outlets for built-up emotions

- **Environmental self-care:** decluttering your home, workspace, organizing documents, making lists, creating a calming area in your home

• **Financial self-care:** taking care of debt, saving, keeping track of your budget, learning about investments

• **Social self-care:** ending relationships with people who encourage toxicity, building a support system

• **Recreational self-care:** traveling, enjoying a good movie/series, spending time in nature, doing puzzles or creative activities

• **Spiritual self-care:** taking regular time for self-reflection, meditation, mindfulness, breathwork

Don't feel the need to start all of these tips to develop empathy at once. To build strong habits that stick for a lifetime, it's best to commit to a few and then add to them instead of overwhelming yourself with too many at once. Trying to take on too much can cause more stress and distractions! Pick a few that make more sense to you and that genuinely motivate you.

After dedicating significant time to overcoming negativity, fear, and anxiety, it is time to move on to the next chapter and fill the void with positive thoughts and actions.

CHAPTER SEVEN: BYE BYE BAD VIBES

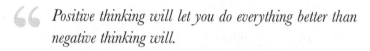 *Positive thinking will let you do everything better than negative thinking will.*

ZIG ZIGLAR

Ziglar's words may seem obvious, but people often overlook the power of the concept. Picture any of the things that you need to do today. I will use ironing as an example because it's certainly not something I love. The process of ironing is going to be the same, no matter what. As always, I have options. I can complain about the ironing, get all grumpy, and ruin the mood of my entire family. Or I can put on a good movie, work my way through the pile, and enjoy the sense of achievement once it's done.

Naturally, the best choice is the latter, but with everything that is going on in our minds and the tendency to lean toward the negative, the positive option isn't going to occur without effort. This is where the C in the REFLECT framework applies, the technique of creating genuine positivity.

WHY SEE THE GLASS HAVE FULL?

The glass half full or half empty is probably the most common metaphor related to positive thinking, and it does actually explain how various people will have different mindsets toward life and experiences. It's not about looking at the world through rose-colored glasses and ignoring the negative aspects of life. It's about being able to think positively about yourself, your abilities, other people, and the challenges you face.

There are several benefits to positive thinking, physical and mental. It's a great way to manage stress levels because positively facing stressful situations can reduce anxiety. Chronic stress and anxiety can increase the risk of diseases such as diabetes, high blood pressure, and heart disease. Positive thinking not only reduces stress levels but also increases immunity to help reduce the risk of illnesses.

In the real world, stress isn't just going to disappear. Those with a pessimistic outlook are going to struggle to handle the ongoing turmoil stress causes. But when you learn how to increase your positivity, you get better at coping with problems, and therefore, your resilience builds as you fix problems instead of giving up hope.

Positive thinking has a wonderful effect on relationships. It's contagious! Being around someone who looks for positive things can bring more fun, happiness, and enjoyment into the relationship. You can inspire each other to achieve more and help each other through the more challenging times. And this isn't just limited to romantic relationships. Positive thinking can improve relationships with family, friends, and coworkers.

There is something essential that you have to bear in mind with positive thinking—it can't be forced. In today's society, there is a lot of what's called toxic positivity. This is when we tell ourselves or hear messages that there is only room for positivity. We may be scrolling through social media with "Positive vibes only" or a friend telling us "It could be worse." You may have even heard yourself using phrases like "Look on the bright side" or "Think happy thoughts."

On the outside, things could be worse, but there might be a bright side. These phrases are only attempts to reassure, but toxic positivity tends to cover or bury the negative instead of accepting it. It can leave people feeling like their problems or perceived negative emotions aren't valid, despite seeing how all emotions are valid, and everyone has the right to express their emotions.

In the case of ironing, toxic positivity would mean ignoring my dread of such a tedious task and forcing myself to smile through the mountain. Suppressing thoughts and feelings often only leads to them resurfacing and becoming more assertive. My negative thoughts would only make them worse. Genuine positivity is accepting that ironing is not a task I enjoy but one that is essential and will make me feel better once it's done.

What many people forget is that whether the glass is half full or half empty, it can always be refilled!

ARE YOU A NEGATIVITY NANCY OR NEGATIVE NED?

To an extent, we are all negative Nancys or negative Neds. Our brains are hard-wired this way as a survival technique. Cavemen had to err on the side of caution and assume a rustle in the bushes was a sign of danger. If not, they may have found themselves as a predator's next meal. Although humans have evolved and don't face the same dangers as in the past, the basic need to stay safe still encourages us to err on the side of caution.

In Chapter 4, we began to understand cognitive distortions, focusing on catastrophizing. Now, it's time to discover other tendencies to lean toward negative thinking.

• **Filtering:** In a situation where there are positives and negatives, you tend to filter the positives and only focus on the negatives.

• **Discounting the positive:** This is another type of filtering, but in this case, when you think of a positive, you dismiss its value.

• **Polarization:** This all-or-nothing thinking causes you to think in black and white. You may end up with unrealistic standards, lack of motivation, and/or setting yourself up for failure.

- **Overgeneralization:** One isolated event becomes a pattern of defeat, often combined with words like always and never, for example, saying "I always mess up" after one mistake.

- **Jumping to conclusions:** There is a situation, and without evidence to support your thoughts, you assume the worst and then react based on the assumption.

- **Personalization:** Taking everything to heart and taking responsibility for everything, even things that are out of your control.

- **Emotional reasoning:** An emotional reaction you experience proves something is real or true, but there is no evidence to support this.

- **Shoulds:** Should statements are based on rules we set for ourselves about how things "should" go a certain way. When things don't go as expected, even if the rules are unreasonable, it's easy to become disappointed, frustrated, or guilty.

- **Labeling:** Placing negative labels on yourself and/or others, including when there is no reason for them. These labels end up attacking a person's character rather than their one-off actions.

- **Always being right:** Nobody likes being wrong, but the need to always be right becomes a cognitive distortion when you go to great lengths to prove your point.

Chapter 4 also covered cognitive reconstructing and the five steps to reframe negative thoughts for more realistic and positive thoughts. The same steps can be used for any type of cognitive distortion. However, take some extra time to identify which type of cognitive distortion your negative thought is. The better you know your thought patterns, the easier it is to spot triggers and make changes.

These cognitive distortions feed the inner critic, and before you know it, negative self-talk takes over. You need to be accountable for your less than ideal behavior, but at the same time, you are committed to improving and should show yourself some self-compassion. Some of your actions may not have been the best choices, but that doesn't mean you're not intelligent! Be kind to yourself. If self-compassion doesn't come easy, imagine a loved one in the same position as you. What would you say to them? You might say to a friend, "That was stupid," but you would never tell them that they are stupid. Have the same compassion for yourself.

If the distorted thought continues to appear despite attempts at reframing, it's time to delve deeper into why. Ask yourself if this thought is bringing you any benefits and if it will help you become the person you want to be. Or is it just going to continue to cause you pain?

For additional help identifying and modifying cognitive distortions, you can use Socratic questioning. Named after the great thinker himself, Socratic questioning is a series of open-ended questions that pushes you beyond your comfort zone and increases your perspective. Use the following questions to further challenge your cognitive distortions:

- What is the problem?

- Why is this problem significant?

- What assumptions have you made?

- Can a different assumption be made?

- What would an outsider think about this problem?

- How would an outsider respond to this problem?

- How can you rephrase the problem for clarification?

- What has led you to your beliefs?

- What additional information do you need?

- What evidence supports your beliefs?

- What reasons do you have to doubt the evidence?

- What evidence are you ignoring?

- Finally, is this the worst-case scenario or not?

Imagine your Socratic questioning as an interview between yourself and yourself in the third person. Each question should provide you with the opportunity for a follow-up question (one of the above or others that are specific to your situation) so that you can learn more about your thoughts.

Just because negative thoughts can become manageable, it doesn't mean that life is automatically full of joy and positivity. In the final section of this chapter, we will cover ways to embrace a positive lifestyle without making it toxic!

TURNING FROWNS UPSIDE DOWN

Chris wasn't a negative person, but he wasn't a positive person either. He felt like he was just floating through life with a solid routine. He worked, paid the bills, and kept fit and healthy. However, nothing he did made him feel enthusiastic, happy, or excited. Looking through an old photo album with his sister, he saw a picture of them horse riding as children. The image reminded him of how much he enjoyed horse riding, and he decided to take up his old hobby again. It was only one hour every couple of weeks, but it was enough to change his outlook on life.

So many things that contribute to positivity are subjective, including love, happiness, hope, and levels of satisfaction. What will bring satisfaction into your life can differ significantly from the next person. What we all have in common is that we deserve some time to ourselves for the things we enjoy in life. This isn't the same as being self-centered because you aren't constantly putting your needs above the needs of others. It's an act of self-care that ensures you are mentally looking after yourself so that you are in a better position to care for others.

If you had one hour a week where you had no responsibilities or obligations, what would you do to bring happiness and positivity into your life? Don't just think about it, make it happen!

Two daily practices that take only a few minutes and

have been scientifically proven to increase positivity are gratitude and positive affirmations.

Gratitude

Once a year, many of us take the time to give thanks for what we have; however, this is just a snapshot of gratitude, and we miss out on all the benefits on the other 364 days of the year.

One study on gratitude involved three groups of people. One group was asked to write a few sentences each week about situations that had occurred and made them feel grateful. The next group was asked to write about things that had annoyed or irritated them and the third group was asked to write about things that had happened without any emphasis on how the events made them feel.

After ten weeks, the group that wrote about what made them feel grateful was more optimistic, felt better about their lives, and even had fewer doctor's visits than the group that had focused on the negatives (Harvard Health Publishing, 2021).

There are two sides to gratitude. On the one hand, a state of gratitude is about acknowledging that life is good and there are things worth living for. On the other hand, gratitude is also about recognizing that there are external sources of goodness in life beyond what comes from within. The source of that goodness can come from other people, nature, actions, or anything else in the world that adds to this goodness of life.

It's not just about people who go out of their way to do something for you. Recently, I was talking to someone who lives in the UK, and they told me that within the last seven months, there had only been four days without rain. At that moment, I felt grateful for the sun on my face! Gratitude is often about the simple, everyday pleasures that are all too often overlooked or unnoticed.

Here are some activities you can try to start practicing gratitude:

- **Rapid-fire gratitude:** You have one minute to list ten things you are grateful for. Try to combine this with mindful gratitude and list things that you are grateful for in the present moment.

- **Gratitude journaling:** Spend a few minutes a day writing about what you are grateful for in your life and why.

- **A gratitude jar:** Every day, write what you are grateful for on a small slip of paper and place it inside a jar. When the jar is full, look back and read all the slips.

- **A gratitude board:** Use photos, images, quotes, or anything that reminds you of things you are grateful for. Keep your board in a place where you can see it frequently.

- **A gratitude walk:** Go for a mindful walk and make a mental note of all the things you are grateful for along the way. Use all five of your senses to tune into nature.

- **Sharing your gratitude:** Write letters or simple

Post-it notes to let others know how grateful you are to have them in your life.

Positive Affirmations

Positive affirmations are short phrases that are repeated to cultivate a positive mental attitude. Science has shown that these affirmations can improve education, health, and relationships. These phrases can create a positive feedback loop that leads to lasting positive effects (Cohen & Sherman, 2014).

Understanding how positive affirmations work has become simpler, thanks to neuroplasticity. Previously, negative thoughts that were replayed in the mind created strong neuro connections that were easy to retrieve. As soon as these thoughts weren't repeated, the connections started to get weaker during the synapse pruning stage. The first time a positive affirmation is said, a new neuro connection is created, and with repetition, the connection becomes stronger.

For positive affirmations to work, you have to truly believe in the words you are repeating. So, it's important that you choose affirmations that you can relate to and feel comfortable saying. That's not to say that the affirmations have to be true. Phrases such as "I love myself" or "I am confident" may not reflect your current state, but by telling your brain this, you will change your way of thinking, and soon enough, you will love yourself and be confident.

Here are some more examples of positive affirmations:

- I am enough

- I am a good person

- I trust myself

- I am stronger than my fears

- I am capable

- I choose to focus on the positive

- I am open to receiving love

- I am worthy of joy and happiness

- I let go of fear and embrace healing

- I allow myself to make mistakes and learn from them

- I am safe

- I am in the right place and going in the right direction

Feel free to change, combine, or write your own affirmations. Just remember to use the present tense and avoid all negative words (e.g., never) and negative contractions (e.g., don't).

Positive affirmations can be used at any time of the day, but they will be especially useful in times of high stress. If you feel the physical symptoms burning up inside you, take a few deep breaths and use your go-to positive affirmation.

Increasing positivity doesn't mean there won't be difficult moments in the future. It's the tough times in life when self-care should also become more of a priority. Take extra time for self-reflection to understand what your mind and body need and then fulfill those needs.

Finally, when the going gets tough, spend time with those who are filled with positivity. Just like other people's negativity can rub off on you, so can positivity. While you may think that this is the time you need to hold on to your own positivity as much as possible, sharing it with others can boost your happiness; after all, your glass is refillable!

Rome wasn't built in a day, and considering you might be tackling toxic behaviors that you have been dealing with for a long time, you are going to need to be patient with yourself. In our final chapter, we will see how that is possible!

CHAPTER EIGHT: SLOW AND STEADY

 The road to success is always under construction.

LILY TOMLIN

It's only natural to want to see instant change. You have worked hard to understand your behaviors, and it's been painful to accept how these behaviors have impacted the lives of your loved ones.

It can even be frustrating that you haven't reached the best version of yourself yet.

At this stage, it's crucial not to let frustration undo the progress and revert to old habits. The final stage of the REFLECT framework will show you how to trust the process!

PATIENCE IN TRANSFORMATION

Life is often focused on getting from point A to point B, but then we realize it's not that simple. We break things down and aim to get from A to Z. Right when we are about to reach Z, something happens that throws us off course. This is because the goal is only the destination, and we overlook the journey process.

Personal growth isn't something you achieve after a certain amount of time or a number of steps. You won't wake up one morning and think, "That's it, I've achieved personal growth." It should be something that you wake up and experience every morning.

The transformation you hope to achieve takes time and patience. But it's not all about you. You will have to extend your patience to those you have hurt in the past. You may have promised change before, only to continue with the same toxic traits. Your loved ones have fallen for empty promises in the past and are going to be cautious about trusting you this time.

Just as you can't rush or force your own change, you can't rush or force them into forgiving you and moving forward.

We live in a world where instant gratification is the norm, so patience is increasingly difficult. The root cause of impatience is frustration, especially when you feel like your needs and wishes aren't being met. This often gives stress, anxiety, and anger a chance to surface. However, patience is a skill that can be learned.

The first step to patience is mindfulness and embracing the present moment. The journey you are on will involve continuous change and growth. This means your thoughts and emotions won't remain the same, your values and beliefs may grow with you, and all of these changing circumstances can mean you aren't always in tune with who you are and where you are going.

Get good at sitting and being comfortable with the present moment. Put down the technology, ignore the to-do list for a moment, and just sit with your feelings. Sometimes, these feelings will bring you great joy. Gratitude mindfulness is about tuning into your senses, focusing on your breath, and contemplating all the things you are grateful for.

Other times, mindful moments can bring up feelings of discomfort. Impatience is especially uncomfortable because mindfulness can feel like you are doing nothing, and if you are doing nothing, how can you possibly be making steps toward your goals?

Use mindfulness as a chance to get good at sitting with feelings of discomfort. Even after you mend broken bridges and increase positivity in your life, there will still be challenging times ahead, leading to inevitable uncomfortable feelings. Start with short periods of discomfort and gradually expose yourself to longer amounts.

Mindfulness can also give you a chance to practice acceptance. Just like uncomfortable feelings, there will be unpleasant situations ahead, and some will test your patience. Acceptance isn't about giving up and not attempting to change things. It's about realizing that there are moments when change is not within your control. This can be any situation, from being stuck in traffic to giving your partner space and time to heal. Focus on what is in your control, like using this time in traffic for deep breathing and mindfulness or committing to showing your partner that this time, it's for real.

Great news for those of us who find waiting a challenge! Learning to resist the temptation of instant gratification is definitely possible—no fate or destiny involved. According to fresh looks at the iconic Marshmallow Experiment, there's hope for everyone to master the art of patience.

In the 1960s, Professor Walter Mischel conducted the marshmallow experiment on a group of 4- and 5-year-olds. Each child was offered a choice: one marshmallow now or two marshmallows later. One marshmallow was left on the table, and the adult left the room for 15 minutes. Some children barely waited until the door was closed, but others made it to the full 15 minutes (Clear, n.d.).

Recent studies give us more insights. It turns out, a child's ability to hold off for the extra marshmallow can be shaped by many factors—like their background, how much they trust the marshmallow-promiser, and their past experiences.

This suggests that with the right environment and guidance, anyone can boost their self-control muscles. So, if you ever felt bad about not passing the Marshmallow Test, cheer up! Delaying gratification isn't a fixed trait— it's a skill we can all develop with a little practice (and maybe a few marshmallows along the way).

Delayed gratification may not be related to freeing yourself from toxic traits, but it will help you develop more patience. Try it with a few simple examples first. For example, instead of a reward after completing each task on your to-do list, think of a bigger reward once you have finished two or three items.

Don't forget that right now, you are growing, even if it doesn't feel like it. Each page you read gives you knowledge and chances to practice newly acquired skills. Instead of chasing the dream, enjoy this moment and rest assured that you are exactly where you should be!

POTENTIAL BUMPS ALONG THE ROAD

If personal growth and transformation were easy, we would all be doing it! Some people never start, while others start and give up at the first obstacle. Others are more realistic and don't expect instant results but soon give up when they don't see the results as quickly as they had hoped.

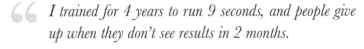 *I trained for 4 years to run 9 seconds, and people give up when they don't see results in 2 months.*

USAIN BOLT

Success requires patience and determination, but certain beliefs can get in the way of both. One of the worst is the assumption that change happens automatically. Reading this book is like following a recipe. Unless you actually follow the recipe steps, you won't get the desired meal outcome. Knowledge will only take you so far and your growth depends on you actively using the skills you have learned on a regular basis. On a similar note, don't wait for the right time! Yes, you have a lot on your plate, but you will still have all the same responsibilities next week and probably next month. The longer you wait to start, the greater the risk of never getting around to it.

Two other beliefs to get past are the perfection belief and the fear of mistakes. You may find yourself asking what the best way to start your personal growth is, more so if your toxic traits have affected multiple people.

There is no perfect way to start because there is no such thing as perfection. Spending time on such a question leads to procrastination, and once again, you may never begin. This takes us to the fact that mistakes will be made.

Accept that personal growth can be messy, and you may have moments when your behavior resembles past toxic traits. That's not to say that you are your old self and haven't made any progress. Those around you will notice you are going in the right direction and understand setbacks, but they may not accept you giving up at the first sign of challenges.

TRUSTING THE PROCESS

Why should you place your trust in such an intangible process? Firstly, it's another part of acceptance. There is no magic pill that is going to enable you to overcome your toxic traits, and although this might sound depressing, it's actually inspiring. Certain things are out of your control, but your personal growth isn't one of them, as long as you persevere in those smaller steps.

Life will throw curveballs and there won't be a magic pill to fix these curveballs either. This is why you need to have faith in your abilities and know that you have what it takes to overcome everything that comes flying your way. You may need some extra information or new skills to do so, but with patience and time, you will get there.

Having trust in the process is good for your health. How many times have you stressed about things not going according to your plan, most likely because you are focusing on the result and not how you are going to get there?

Knowing that you will get there takes away this stress and replaces it with positivity and optimism. Isn't it better to know that you will achieve what you want in a month or in a year than never at all?

Part of trusting the process is to remind yourself to be patient. However, it's also about having the right mindset, and in this case, it will require a growth mindset. A fixed mindset is where you believe your abilities and skills are fixed and there is no room for improvement. A growth mindset embraces challenges, focusing on progress instead of the end result. The growth mindset is supported by neuroplasticity because the fact that we can't learn new things past a certain age is now a myth.

The word "can't" is detrimental to the growth mindset. Imagine if one trait you want to overcome is your temper. For six days of the week, you have controlled your temper, but on the seventh day, you lose it. Cognitive distortions kick in, and you tell yourself that you will never be able to control your temper despite the evidence presented in the last few days.

Rather than saying, "I can't control my temper," change the sentence to "I can't control my temper yet." By simply adding the word "yet" to the end of the sentence, you are telling yourself that you are trusting the process and it will happen.

For those dark times when you lack faith in both yourself and the process, turn to your loved ones for inspiration. Remind yourself why they are so amazing and a crucial part of your life.

> *If you can remember why you started, then you will know why you must continue.*
>
> ### CHRIS BURKMENN

Now that you are growing and overcoming your toxic flaws, your friends and family deserve the opportunity to see what a wonderful and caring person you really arc.

While the road to success may always be under construction, never forget that you are the builder. You have the tools to build that road, and more importantly, you have the ability to choose which direction you build that road!

CONCLUSION

What a journey it has been so far! At the beginning of this book, it's likely you knew something wasn't quite right, but you couldn't exactly put your finger on what that was. You experienced strain and tension in your relationships, but if you were completely honest with yourself, you may not have fully realized the extent of your role in this.

It's an unpleasant experience reflecting on your own flaws and how this has caused such suffering for those you love. I commend you for doing this, and you should be proud of yourself. Many wouldn't make the effort to do the same and would continue leading a life that ignores the needs of others.

The point of self-reflection and discovering more about yourself wasn't to make you feel bad about who you are. Instead, it was the first step toward identifying the root cause of your toxic behavior. That's not to say you can blame your past and not hold yourself accountable. It was a chance for you to understand that apparent anger, frustration, and contempt are actually caused by deep-seated fears of inadequacy and low self-esteem. Whether your biggest fear is showing your vulnerable side or being abandoned, you need to overcome these fears if you want to leave your toxic traits in the past.

When you start working on yourself, you are laying the foundations for a clean slate. This is when you can begin to understand how your communication has built a wall between you and meaningful connections with others. Toxic behaviors aren't just physical and verbal abuse; they can also be not listening to people or constantly interrupting them. You laid the foundations, and now it's time to build bridges through nonviolent communication that doesn't involve any form of manipulation, intentional or not. Don't forget the importance of a genuine, heartfelt apology when building bridges.

Picture a world where everyone has the ability to take on other people's perspectives and then take that to the next level and actually feel the pain and suffering of others. As we take baby steps, let's work on your ability to empathize with those around you. A lack of empathy often stems from differences and an inability to respect the fact that we are all entitled to our individual beliefs, values, and thoughts. Ironically, to close these gaps, you need to accept that people are different and then look for common ground. It's the similarities you share with others that will allow you to share how a person feels, both their joys and sorrows.

It would also be nice to picture a more positive world, but this is out of your control. What you are accountable for is your own positivity. Cognitive reframing will help prune out those automatic negative thoughts, and then practicing things like gratitude and positive affirmations will create new neuro connections that can strengthen with time and regular practice.

The REFLECT framework is *a* process for you to trust, as it will guide you through the beginning of your transformation. Here's a recap:

- **R:** recognize toxic traits

- **E:** explore perspectives

- **F:** face your fears

- **L:** learn healthy patterns of interaction

- **E:** empathize with others

- **C:** cultivate positivity

- **T:** trust the process

Nevertheless, this isn't *the* process, as my friend Simon quickly discovered. Simon had pretty much ruined his relationship with his brother. It started in high school with some healthy competition but escalated to ridiculous levels. Simon went out of his way to get one up on his brother. He would purposely wait until his brother bought a car so that he could buy a better one. He also bought a bigger house than his brother despite not needing it and putting himself in financial trouble. Additionally, he would choose girlfriends that give him a reason to show off than women he actually liked. His brother didn't retaliate, but they grew further and further apart. After several failed relationships, Simon soon realized that he needed his older brother in his life and began the REFLECT process.

Unfortunately, Simon focused on the A to B, and after making amends with his brother, he felt that he had achieved his goal. But old patterns started to resurface, and by the time their father passed away, the brothers were once again not speaking. Now more than ever, Simon needed a relationship with his brother, so he began the process again, but this time, he accepted that this wouldn't be achieved overnight. Instead, he knew it was something he would have to continue to work on.

This change in Simon's mindset opened more doors than he could ever imagine. He now rents his brother's annex, and they have weekly game nights where they can put aside the notion that men don't have feelings and talk openly and honestly. Simon's finances are back on track, and he is now in a position to put down a deposit on a house with his girlfriend, a woman he admires and respects. At the same time, he knows that while this is success and a reason to celebrate, there is more to his journey and his unique process.

Change is scary. It's the unknown and the unpredictable. Your mind might be tempted to focus on everything that could go wrong, but you have the wisdom and the tools to embrace this much-needed change. It won't be instant, but it will happen if you start today with small, manageable, and consistent steps.

I have one last thing to ask of you. Considering the misuse of the word narcissist, there are so many people walking around in life, maybe even those you know, who are suffering from toxic traits but want to overcome them. There is a way you can help them without attempting the impossible and changing the world. By sharing your opinions of this book on Amazon, you can let others know that they can also find their own process to freeing themselves from toxic traits and leading a more positive, connected life. It will only take a 30 seconds, but it can change someone's life who was once in the same situation as you.

Thank you in advance, and rather than wishing you luck, I hope you thrive in the new life that lies ahead of you!

SUMMARY GUIDE

A SHORT MESSAGE FROM THE AUTHOR

I hope you're enjoying the book so far! I have a tiny favor to ask that could make a huge difference. If you could take just 30 seconds to leave a review on Amazon, I would be incredibly grateful.

Reviews are super important for authors—they help us get noticed and keep doing what we love. Yet, they're surprisingly hard to come by!

If you've got a moment to spare and some thoughts to share, I'd love to hear what you think. Even a few words would mean the world to me.

Just scan the QR code on the left to leave a review.

INTRODUCTION

We began by examining what sets you apart from a full-blown narcissist and clarified that even if you have toxic behaviors, you should not label yourself as a narcissist since they will seldom see an error in their ways and rarely seek help.

The truth is, to some degree, we all have moments when toxic traits rise up, which includes falling into the habit of manipulating others. There is still a difference between being an imperfect human and being a bad person.

It's not easy admitting you are wrong or owning up to your flaws. It's even harder when these behaviors come from deep-rooted fears and years of listening to your inner critic. To overcome toxic behaviors and put negativity behind you, it's essential to make a commitment to continuous improvement and recognize that this is going to take time.

Before implementing behavior-changing techniques, the first step is to take a closer look at yourself and why you have reached the point where you are at today.

CHAPTER ONE: MORE THAN JUST VANITY

Though there are different types of narcissism, most commonly, there are overt and covert narcissists.

Overt narcissist traits are what we are more commonly exposed to in the media, so it's normal that this is the impression we have of this personality trait. Overt narcissists are highly outgoing, charismatic, and have a sense of entitlement. These consider themselves to be more intelligent, better looking, and even have good emotional intelligence compared to others. They need to be the center of attention, in contrast to covert narcissists who are often introverted.

Covert narcissists may play the victim to get what they want, and they may become extremely defensive when faced with criticism.

The likelihood of you having narcissistic personality disorder (NPD) is very low. That's not to say that narcissistic traits aren't also seen in other types of disorders, such as borderline personality disorder and post-traumatic stress. If you are concerned, you should talk to a doctor.

The roots of narcissistic behavior can't be exactly pinpointed and may even be a combination of nature and nurture. Brain scans have shown differences in those with NPD and those who don't have it. On the other hand, our childhood experiences, the environment we grew up in, and even past experiences in adulthood can cause toxic traits. Regardless of the roots of your behavior, it's essential that you take responsibility for your emotions, thoughts, and actions.

Fortunately, thanks to neuroplasticity and the brain's ability to adapt to changing environments, we now know that it is possible to break free from negative and toxic traits and make way for more positive interactions with yourself and others.

This is when we introduce the **REFLECT** framework:

- **R:** recognize toxic traits

- **E:** explore perspectives

- **F:** face your fears

- **L:** learn healthy patterns of interaction

- **E:** empathize with others

- **C:** cultivate positivity

- **T:** trust the process

It's this framework that will guide us through the following chapters and the process of change.

Here is a recap of the key points in chapter one:

- Narcissism is a highly complex personality disorder that goes beyond an inflated sense of self.

- You have narcissistic traits, not NPD, or else you wouldn't be reading this book.

- Nobody knows the exact cause of narcissism, but it's likely a combination of nature and nurture.

- Narcissistic traits can cause immense emotional turmoil, affecting your mental health, the mental health of those around you, and society as a whole.

- Thanks to neuroplasticity, your brain can change, and

you can replace negative aspects of your life with positive experiences.

CHAPTER TWO: RED FLAG ALERTS

For many, this is the hardest part of the process because it requires an honest look at all the ways you have caused your loved ones emotional harm. As you have probably gone through life with little to no self-awareness, you may not even realize that some behaviors are toxic or the extent of the damage they can do. Some of the most common toxic traits include:

- Lying and insincerity

- People pleasing

- Perfectionism

- Flexibility and inflexibility

- Judging others

- Competition

- Negative self-talk

- Pessimism

- Attention-seeking

- Manipulation

- Gaslighting

- Playing the victim

- Guilt-tripping

- The dramatics

- Holding on to the past

- Conversation hogger

- Clinging

- Control freak

- Apathy

- Greed

- Love bombing

There is a process for taking responsibility. It starts by identifying your negative traits and then imagining yourself as a bystander to see exactly what your negative traits look like from the outside. Next, you need to consider the impact these traits have on others and monitor each time these traits arise and precisely what happens in each experience. This doesn't sound like a quick fix, and that's because there is no such thing, but it will increase your awareness.

Though it's hard to hear from others, if you are really struggling to understand the depths of your toxic behaviors, it's a good idea to ask for feedback from someone you trust, as they will be able to highlight issues that are stuck in your blind spot.

Here is a quick recap before we move on to the next stage of the REFLECT framework:

- Toxic traits are anything that causes ongoing distress or

harm to yourself or others; it's not the same as isolated incidents.

• Toxic traits are subjective, meaning that the same negative behavior can impact different people differently.

• The first step to overcoming your toxic traits is to identify them and take responsibility for them.

• Get better at sharing and asking for feedback to discover more about yourself.

• Having toxic traits doesn't make you inherently bad. Pay attention to both the good and the not-so-good feedback that people give you. This is a process, so be kind to yourself!

CHAPTER THREE: LIFE IN HD

Perspective is powerful and determines how we view the world. It is influenced by various factors, such as education, age, mood, personal beliefs, and the media. We saw how one simple image can be seen as a number or a letter depending on the information we have been previously told or shown. Perspectives can also be influenced by bias and the judgments we make of others.

We are now aware of the need for greater diversity and the benefits this brings. However, modern technology isn't helping. Personalized content means that when you search for one thing, a ton of recommendations will come up based on your search. This leads to limited opportunities for exploring other perspectives.

At this point, we aren't attempting to understand a person's emotions in different situations. For now, it's about seeing things as another person would. A classic example is how parents can influence their children based on their own beliefs. If a child sees a parent reading a book, they are more likely to pick up a book. If they see a parent on a tablet, they will want the tablet.

We reviewed five different ways to see things from diverse perspectives, from practicing with fictional characters to real-life situations. In each case, this is a practice that you will need to get into a habit of because, with so many influences, there are an endless number of perspectives you can take on, each bringing new benefits.

Here's a recap of what was covered in this chapter:

• Your perspective is the way you view the world, and it will be unique.

• Perspectives are influenced by a number of factors, especially past experiences.

• Looking at things from different perspectives can increase empathy, problem-solving, and creativity.

• Seeing things from other people's points of view requires a deliberate activation of perspective-taking, unlike our perspectives, which are formed rapidly and automatically.

• Start practicing perspective taking with fictional characters and people you don't know so that your emotional attachments and thoughts don't influence your ability to step into their shoes.

CHAPTER FOUR: FACE THE MUSIC

The third stage of the REFLECT framework explored fears in depth, starting with what happens in both the brain and the body when we are faced with fear. While the hippocampus helps us discern between real and imagined threats, perceived threats, like those that stem from thoughts and emotions rather than visual stimuli, can still cause the body to react in the same way.

There are a great number of fears, and each person may have very different triggers. For some, the fear of being alone is too much to cope with. For others, the need to be in control forces them to become overly controlling, to the point of being overbearing.

Most people experience the fear of failure at some point, but not everyone fears expressing their gratitude as a sign of weakness.

Visualization is a good place to start, as this can ensure that you are mentally and physically calm for the challenge ahead. Gradual exposure breaks down fears into smaller steps.

Once you can face the smallest fear and not have a physical or emotional response, you can move on to the next stage. It's necessary to follow the steps and take your time to succeed with gradual exposure.

Facing fears isn't going to be easy, and you may sometimes feel like you are taking a step back before moving forward. Don't feel you have to do this alone.

Sometimes having a supportive friend nearby can help you, especially when it comes to taking the first step.

Here is our recap for facing fears!

• Fear is an emotion that can cause terrifying symptoms, but fear itself cannot hurt you.

• Some toxic behaviors are related to more obvious fears (like pushing others away to protect yourself from potential rejection), while others are more complex and require deep self-reflection to fully understand.

• Facing fears has to start with a calm mind and the ability to manage physical symptoms.

• Techniques such as gradual exposure and cognitive restructuring are processes that require patience, practice, and time.

• Mindful meditation and journaling are excellent exercises to help overcome fears and also improve mental and physical well-being, especially when done regularly.

CHAPTER FIVE: A NEW LEAF

Chapter two may have seemed like enough self-reflection to understand your toxic behavior and that your self-esteem can't possibly take any more. Understanding negative traits isn't about further attacking you as a person. Much like toxic traits, if you aren't aware of the problem, you won't know where to begin to fix it!

Poor communication can be anything from not listening or paying attention to interrupting, complaining, and stonewalling. At the extreme end of the scale, there is gaslighting, where your words cause another person to doubt their reality. When communication becomes toxic, even the tiniest problems can turn into full-blown arguments.

After a sincere apology, it's time to adopt nonviolent communication. This involves four steps: observations, emotions, needs, and requests. Using this structure can make it clear that you are communicating your emotions rather than how another person has made you feel, an act of accountability, and it makes it clear what changes you would like to see. It's a perfect example of being assertive and ensuring the other person doesn't feel attacked or disrespected.

As you are using the structure for nonviolent communication highlighted in this chapter, don't forget to combine it with the HONEST acronym to steer you away from passive-aggressive and aggressive communication:

Hold your ground

Open-mindedness

Nonverbal cues

Express yourself clearly

Self-awareness

Take responsibility.

Here is our recap to turning over that new leaf:

• Journal to identify your negative behavior patterns, understand your triggers, and think about the consequences.

• Make a heartfelt apology, preferably face-to-face, to those you have hurt, but don't forget it's up to them whether they choose to forgive you.

• Follow the four steps to nonviolent communication and practice sentences with less than 50 words.

• Manipulation isn't always bad or intentional, but it can be extremely painful for those on the receiving end. Before you can stop manipulating others, you have to recognize when you are doing it!

• Improving self-esteem, communication and boundaries are strategies to stop manipulating others—but you have to be accountable!

CHAPTER SIX: HEART WIDE OPEN

Empathy is the next step in perspective taking. Now that you can see things from different points of view, you will find it easier to take on people's emotions in various situations—the art of empathy!

There are three types of empathy. Affective empathy is the ability to respond to other people's emotions appropriately, somatic empathy is when you can genuinely feel what someone else is feeling, and cognitive empathy is when you can understand why people have certain emotional reactions to situations.

To be blunt, regardless of whether you have narcissistic traits or narcissistic personality disorder, you still can show empathy. You might just lack the motivation. There might be barriers to empathy, such as cognitive biases, fear, and stress, but all of these can be overcome with the right mindset and willingness.

Common ground may feel like the opposite of seeking different opinions. After all, to appreciate perspectives, you need to look for people and experiences separate from what you are usually exposed to. Common ground is about looking for similarities. The trick is to step out of your comfort zone enough to expose yourself to the differences, ask open-ended questions to discover more, and then respect the fact that others may not share your beliefs.

As we reach the end of the E in the REFLECT framework, it's time for our recap:

• Empathy is the ability to connect with others on an emotional level and to feel what they are feeling.

• Narcissists are labeled as having no empathy, but that's not the case. It's a skill anyone can learn if they are motivated to.

• Barriers to empathy, including dehumanization, fear, victim blaming and distractions can be overcome with greater self-awareness.

• Begin to improve self-awareness by banning overused words that don't accurately label your emotions and use the list to choose more appropriate ones.

- To empathize with others, you need to step past your normal experiences so that you can put yourselves in the same uncomfortable positions that others go through.

- When someone chooses you to share their words and feelings, recognize your importance in their life and respect them by listening with your heart and your head, regardless of the stress and problems you are dealing with.

CHAPTER SEVEN: BYE BYE BAD VIBES

Although cognitive restructuring was introduced as a technique to overcome negative thoughts related to fears in chapter four, this is the chapter that really delved into cognitive distortions and our tendency to lean toward the negative. While working through the steps to reframing automatic negative thoughts, consider if these cognitive distortions are affecting your thoughts, emotions, and perspective:

- Filtering

- Discounting the positive

- Polarization

- Overgeneralization

- Jumping to conclusions

- Personalization

- Emotional reasoning

- Shoulds

- Labeling

- Always being right

Negative thoughts are sometimes easy to recognize and rephrase, and chapter four will have provided enough guidance for this. For those negative thoughts that just won't give you a moment of peace, it's time to use Socratic questioning. Socratic questioning is a system of open-ended questions that takes you just far enough past your comfort zone to understand the deeper reasons behind your thought patterns.

As we work toward a more positive life, it's crucial that the negatives aren't just masked with superficial positivity. This is one area of life that you can't fake until you make it.

Toxic positivity causes us to ignore or suppress any negativity in our lives in place of forced positivity. Life may be greener on the other side, but that doesn't mean that what you feel right now isn't valid.

Gratitude is a way to bring genuine positivity into your life. Too often, we start by listing things we feel we should be grateful for, such as your family, your partner, or the roof over your head.

Of course, these are reasons to be grateful, but there are also the less obvious reasons in the world that deserve gratitude, many of which are personal. I am grateful for the 45 minutes of *Grey's Anatomy*, where I curl up on the sofa with my daughter and ignore my phone!

In this chapter, we also looked at positive affirmations as a way to rewire the brain's habit of negative thinking. Disney has, in the past, created some unrealistic expectations and affirmations. Is it really enough to wish upon a star?

Fortunately, the company has moved on with the times and we have excellent examples of positive affirmations, for example, "Fairy tales can come true. You've got to make them happen. It all depends on you!"

Let's finish up with our penultimate recap!

• A positive outlook has several mental and physical health benefits, particularly, stress management and reducing the risk of chronic health conditions, but only when it's genuine.

• Negative thoughts aren't your fault. They are the brain's tendency to look at the glass half empty as a survival mechanism.

• Cognitive reframing can help you with cognitive distortions, but Socratic questioning may give you deeper answers to those persistent thought patterns.

• Gratitude is about recognizing that there is good in you and your life, and there are external contributors, all of which deserve gratitude, even those smaller things that may get overlooked.

• Positive affirmations work by creating new positive neuro connections that get stronger each time they are repeated.

- In times of high stress, make time for your own needs through self-care, being around positivity, and acts of kindness to encourage others to feel more positive.

CHAPTER EIGHT: SLOW AND STEADY

Yes, it may have been a shorter chapter, but it is significant, nonetheless. If you think about the bigger picture, your thoughts and behaviors have developed over time, maybe months, maybe years. You can't possibly expect to change these habits in hours or days.

You are going to need patience, not only with yourself but also with others. And my final piece of harsh advice: you may need more patience with your loved ones than you first thought.

Consider this:

 Insanity is doing the same thing over and over and expecting a different result.

ALBERT EINSTEIN

From the perspective of others, you have to make changes, even if they are gradual, if you want to see a difference in your relationships. It won't be today or tomorrow. But if you trust the fact that this is ongoing personal growth, your loved ones will appreciate the steps you are taking.

The REFLECT framework is *a process* in itself but it's not *the* process.

- Personal growth isn't about getting from A to B; it's a journey that will have ups and downs, but as long as you are dedicated to moving forward, you will continue to grow.

- Such a transformation requires patience with yourself and those around you. Get good at sitting with the discomfort of impatience with the help of mindfulness.

- While you should reward yourself for the progress you make, try delayed gratification every now and then to increase your levels of patience.

- Don't expect everything to happen at once, don't wait for the perfect time, and don't fear the mistakes you will inevitably make. Some obstacles will be out of your control, but these are things you can control.

- Develop a growth mindset and trust the process because even when it doesn't feel like it, you've got this!

CONCLUSION

In Pink's words, "It hurts to be human." It hurts that you may have spotted some aspects of your life, but it hurts more when you consider the impact of these traits. You want to overcome toxic traits, but it hurts more when you realize the extent of your behaviors.

But let's look at an alternative perspective from Pink: "You gotta get up and try, try, try." Online, there are so many steps to get from A to B, but many fail to realize that actual growth isn't about getting to B. It's about recognizing that it's not the A to B or even the A to Z.

Your individual process and progress depend on you committing to small yet consistent changes for tomorrow, the next month, and the years to come! With every small step you master, the lifelong dream becomes more attainable!

———

I HAVE ONE LAST THING TO ASK OF YOU

Considering the misuse of the word narcissist, there are so many people walking around in life, maybe even those you know, who are suffering from toxic traits but want to overcome them. There is a way you can help them without attempting the impossible and changing the world.

By sharing your opinions of this book on Amazon, you can let others know that they can also find their own process to freeing themselves from toxic traits and leading a more positive, connected life. It will only take a 30 seconds, but it can change someone's life who was once in the same situation as you.

Thank you in advance, and rather than wishing you luck, I hope you thrive in the new life that lies ahead of you!

Just scan the QR code on the right to leave a review.

CONTINUE YOUR JOURNEY WITH 'THE ART OF SELF-IMPROVEMENT' SERIES BY CHASE HILL

HOW TO STOP NEGATIVE THINKING

This guide breaks down **seven easy steps to tackle everything from fleeting intrusive thoughts to deep-seated ruminations.** With practical strategies, exercises, and tools, it helps you pinpoint the roots of your negative thoughts and offers proven techniques to calm your mind.

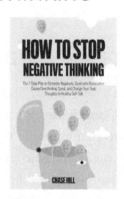

Learn how to **shed toxic behaviors and embrace self-love** and acceptance through positive affirmations and self-talk. If you're ready for a happier, more positive outlook, this guide is your starting point.

HEALTHY BOUNDARIES

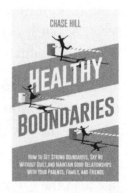

Discover the power of self-love, and learn how to **set healthy boundaries – without feeling guilty**. You don't have to compromise your individuality just to be "considerate" of others. You can set healthy boundaries, and make your friends, family and parents **respect that boundary.**

Setting up boundaries isn't about being rude: it's about acknowledging that **your well-being comes first.** You can start doing what YOU want to do.

SWITCH OFF OVERTHINKING

The modern world fans the flames with its non-stop influx of information, choices to be made, and the pressure to always be switched 'on'. It's no wonder your mind is in overdrive.

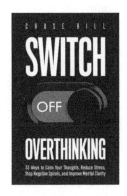

But imagine a toolkit, one that's been tested in the trenches of the busiest of minds, offering **not just quick fixes, but sustainable strategies**.

With over 30 strategies to choose from and apply, you can create your own path toward mental peace, emotional resilience, and serenity.

READY FOR MORE INSIGHTS AND INSPIRATION? SCAN THE QR CODE TO FIND MORE BOOKS BY CHASE HILL AND CONTINUE YOUR JOURNEY.

BIBLIOGRAPHY

"A Quote by Brené Brown." n.d. https://www.goodreads.com/quotes/357565-owning-our-story-can-be-hard-but-not-nearly-as.

"A Quote by Chris Burkmenn." n.d. https://www.goodreads.com/quotes/1301857-if-you-can-remember-why-you-started-then-you-will.

Abram, Tracie. 2013. "Barriers to Empathy." MSU Extension. September 27, 2013. https://www.canr.msu.edu/news/barriers_to_empathy.

Ackerman, Sandra. 1992. "The Development and Shaping of the Brain." Discovering the Brain - NCBI Bookshelf. 1992. https://www.ncbi.nlm.nih.gov/books/NBK234146/.

Ambardar, Sheenie, MD. 2023. "Narcissistic Personality Disorder." Medscape. September 27, 2023. https://emedicine.medscape.com/article/1519417-overview?form=fpf.

Bradberry, T., & Greaves, J. (2009). Emotional Intelligence 2.0. TalentSmart.

Brown, B. (2012). Daring Greatly: How the Courage to Be Vulnerable Transforms the Way We Live, Love, Parent, and Lead. Gotham Books.

Burns, Stephanie. 2021. "What 'Finding Your Why' Really Means." Forbes, May 24, 2021. https://www.forbes.com/sites/stephanieburns/2021/05/24/what-finding-your-why-really-means/?sh=79c242ee73f4.

Caruso, Catherine. 2023. "A New Field of Neuroscience Aims to Map Connections in the Brain." Harvard Medical School. January 19, 2023. https://hms.harvard.edu/news/new-field-neuroscience-aims-map-connections-brain

Clear, James. 2020. "The Marshmallow Experiment and the Power of Delayed Gratification." James Clear. February 4, 2020. https://jamesclear.com/delayed-gratification

Cohen, Geoffrey L., and David K. Sherman. 2014. "The Psychology of Change: Self-Affirmation and Social Psychological Intervention."

Annual Review of Psychology 65 (1): 333–71. https://doi.org/10.1146/annurev-psych-010213-115137.

Diary, A Coach's. n.d. "Week 6 | Every Success Story Has Some Patience." https://acoachsdiary.blogspot.com/2022/02/week-6-every-success-story-has-some.html.

"Disney Affirmations." n.d. Disney in Your Day. https://www.disneyinyourday.com/disney-affirmations/.

"Empathy Quotes." n.d. BrainyQuote. https://www.brainyquote.com/topics/empathy-quotes.

Graham, Sarah. n.d. "Narcissistic Personality Disorder and Brain Structure." Children of Narcissisits. https://childrenofnarcissists.org.uk/narcissistic-personality-disorder-and-brain-structure/

Hanson, R., & Hanson, F. (2018). Resilient: How to Grow an Unshakable Core of Calm, Strength, and Happiness. Harmony.

Harvard Health. 2021. "Giving Thanks Can Make You Happier." August 14, 2021. https://www.health.harvard.edu/healthbeat/giving-thanks-can-make-you-happier.

Lee, Royce J., David Gozal, Emil F. Coccaro, and Jennifer R. Fanning. 2020. "Narcissistic and Borderline Personality Disorders: Relationship With Oxidative Stress." *Journal of Personality Disorders* 34 (Supplement): 6–24. https://doi.org/10.1521/pedi.2020.34.supp.6.

"Lily Tomlin Quotes." n.d. Brainy Quote. https://www.brainyquote.com/quotes/lily_tomlin_379145.

Mcleod, Saul, PhD. 2023. "Perceptual Set in Psychology: Definition & Examples." *Simply Psychology*, June. https://www.simplypsychology.org/perceptual-set.html.

Miller, Joshua D., Donald R. Lynam, Colin Vize, Michael L. Crowe, Chelsea E. Sleep, Jessica L. Maples-Keller, Lauren R. Few, and W. Keith Campbell. 2017. "Vulnerable Narcissism Is (Mostly) a Disorder of Neuroticism." *Journal of Personality* 86 (2): 186–99. https://doi.org/10.1111/jopy.12303.

Mitrokostas, Sophia. 2018. "New Research Suggests That Narcissists Might Be Able to 'learn' Empathy — but There's a Catch." *Business Insider*, August 2, 2018. https://www.businessinsider.com/can-narcissists-learn-empathy-2018-8.

One Planet. n.d. "Rethinking How We Consume." One Planet Network. https://www.oneplanetnetwork.org/programmes/sustainable-lifestyles-education/about.

"P!Nk – Try." n.d. Genius. https://genius.com/P-nk-try-lyrics.

"P!Nk (Ft. Khalid) – Hurts 2B Human." n.d. Genius. https://genius.com/P-nk-hurts-2b-human-lyrics.

"Quote About Perspective | Self Help Daily." 2016. Self Help Daily. February 24, 2016. https://www.selfhelpdaily.com/tag/quote-about-perspective/.

Rosenberg, M. B. (2003). Nonviolent Communication: A Language of Life. PuddleDancer Press.

Razzetti, Gustavo. 2018. "How to Conquer Your Blind Spots." Fearless Culture. March 25, 2018. https://www.fearlessculture.design/blog-posts/how-to-conquer-your-blind-spots.

Ronningstam, E. n.d. "Narcissistic Personality Disorder: Guide for Providers." Mass General Brigham McLean. https://www.mclean-hospital.org/npd-provider-guide#:~:text=NPD%20in%20DSM%2D5,meet%20the%20di-agnosis%20of%20NPD.

Sandberg, S., & Grant, A. (2017). Option B: Facing Adversity, Building Resilience, and Finding Joy. Knopf.

Sohal, Monika, Pavneet Singh, Bhupinder Singh Dhillon, and Harbir Singh Gill. 2022. "Efficacy of Journaling in the Management of Mental Illness: A Systematic Review and Meta-analysis." NIH. March 18, 2022. https://www.ncbi.nlm.nih.gov/pmc/articles/PMC8935176/.

"Steve Pavlina Quote: 'Fear is not your enemy. It is a compass pointing you to the areas where you need to grow.'" n.d. https://quotefancy.com/quote/1526426/Steve-Pavlina-Fear-is-not-your-enemy-It-is-a-compass-pointing-you-to-the-areas-where-you.

"Truman Capote Quotes." n.d. Goodreads. https://www.goodreads.com/quotes/6767721-i-tell-you-my-dear-narcissus-was-no-egoist-he.

U.S. Department of Health and Human Services Office of Minority Health. n.d. "Communication Styles." Think Cultural Health. https://thinkculturalhealth.hhs.gov/assets/pdfs/resource-library/communication-styles.pdf.

Vater, A., and S. Moritz. 2018. "Does a Narcissism Epidemic Exist in Modern Western Societies? Comparing Narcissism and Self-Esteem in East and West Germany." NIH. January 24, 2018. https://www.ncbi.nlm.nih.gov/pmc/articles/PMC5783345/.

Weiss, M. (2018). Healing from Hidden Abuse: A Journey Through the Stages of Recovery from Psychological Abuse. Morgan James Publishing.

Wilczek, Frank, and Quanta Magazine. 2023. "Einstein's Parable of Quantum Insanity." Scientific American. September 23, 2023. https://www.scientificamerican.com/article/einstein-s-parable-of-quantum-insanity/

Winch, G. (2017). Emotional First Aid: Healing Rejection, Guilt, Failure, and Other Everyday Hurts. Plume.

"Zig Ziglar Quotes." n.d. Brainy Quotes. https://www.brainyquote.com/quotes/zig_ziglar_125675.

Made in United States
Orlando, FL
12 September 2024

51408049R00107